40 Fierce Push Up Bar Exercises for a Perfect & Sexy Body

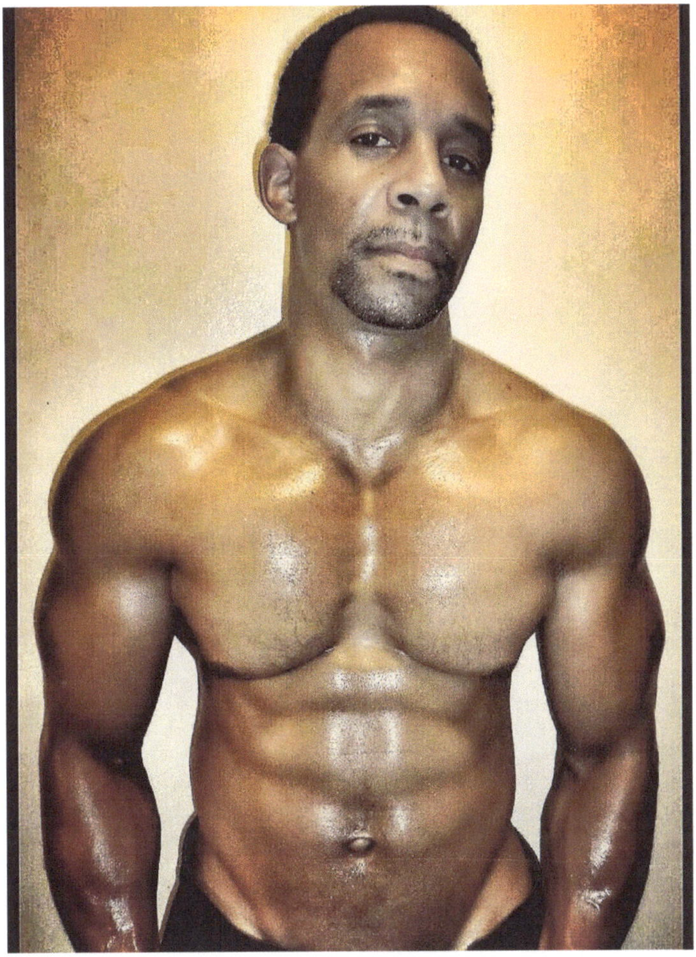

First Printing, 2016

ISBN 1-5305351-2-3

Acknowledgments

I must first start off by thanking my Lord and Savior Jesus Christ for anointing me with His precious Word and Holy Spirit to release my second workout book. Thank you Lord for blessing me and empowering me with your infinite wisdom, revelation knowledge, and understanding to walk by faith and not by sight. With the guidance of your precious Holy Spirit, you allow me to continue to fulfill my godly purpose in life.

Secondly, I would like to give a special shout out to my nephew Christian. He is currently three years old now, and when I talked to his mom (my sister Raquel) on the phone one day, she shares with me one of the greatest inspirational stories I've ever heard. She tells me her and Christian were in the kitchen one night, and she turns around and asks "Christian, what are you doing on the floor?" He responds, "I'm doing pushups like my Uncle Brian!"

Now if that doesn't inspire me, nothing will. Thank you Christian...Uncle Brian loves you.

Table of Contents

Introduction

In the fitness and workout world, ALL men and even most women desire a well-defined, cut, toned, and SEXY chest area to help give their overall upper body that FLAWLESS look. Study shows that on average that women are more attracted to men's chest muscles than any other muscle on their bodies. But in order to get your chest and overall upper body area in tip-top shape, you must first learn how to do the proper exercises.

In general, the standard push up exercise not only works your overall upper body, but it actually activates every muscle in your body. These are the major muscle groups that push up exercises work: chest, triceps, shoulders, and even your core or abdominal areas will get a great workout burn from doing pushups. Now in this book, I've taken your standard push up exercise to a whole new level of intensity by using what is called THE PUSH UP BARS!!

Push up bar exercises are more effective than doing standard push ups with your hands on the floor. They give you a better and more concentrated push up because your body is elevated about 4-6 inches off the floor (depending on the type of bars you have). This will increase your range of motion and in addition to, you will experience less stress and strain on your joints and wrists. Actually the push up bars help maintain your wrists in a neutral position. Now, your forearms will work a little harder to keep your wrists from collapsing. But they keep and maintain your wrists in a safer position throughout the exercise. Also by using the push up bars, your development in these major muscle groups will increase in power and strength by 50-75%.

In this book, I've carefully put together 40 push up bar exercises that will change your fitness life forever. From the how-to, proper form, benefits, and advantages, these push up bar exercises will give your body a good old fashion "shock" to your muscles like never before. Definition, toning, flexibility, and stability in your muscles will increase to an all-time high.

Here are 10 advantages and benefits from using the push up bars:

1. Builds well-defined and toned muscles
2. Increase functional strength
3. Strengthens your core and abdominals
4. Increases flexibility and muscle stretching
5. Enhances your cardiovascular system and increase muscle stamina
6. Helps burn more fat and calories
7. Builds shoulder strength to protect from injury
8. Increases strength in spinal cord and improves posture

9. Engages your muscle more intensively
10. Increased testosterone and reduces osteoporosis development

Each push up bar exercise will be broken down into three detailed categories: Standard (Level 1), Intermediate (Level 2), and Advanced (Level 3).

Let's begin.

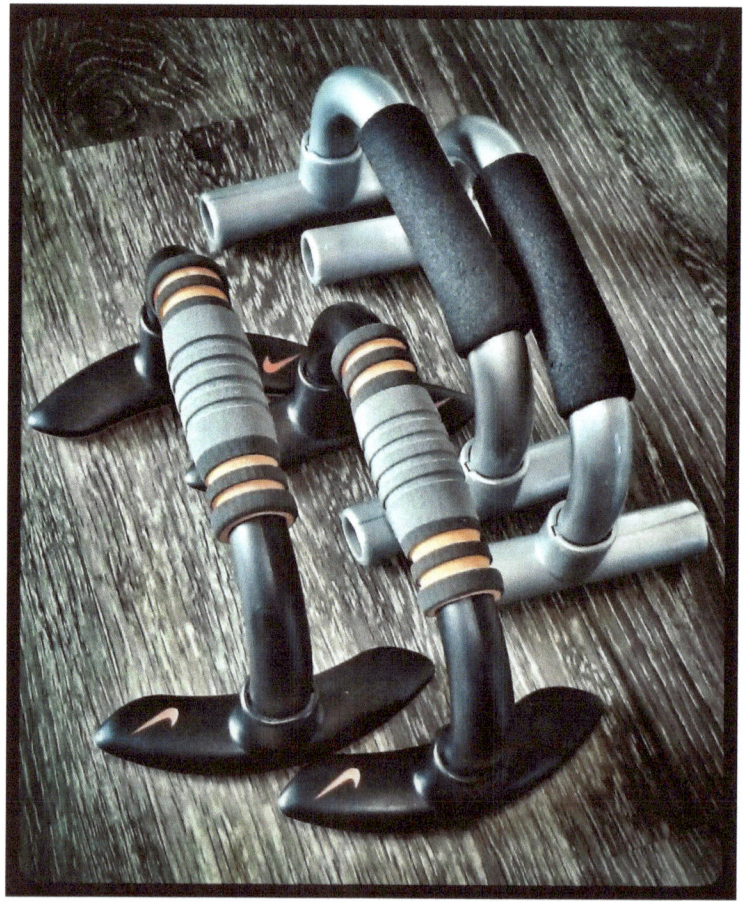

Welcome to the Exercises

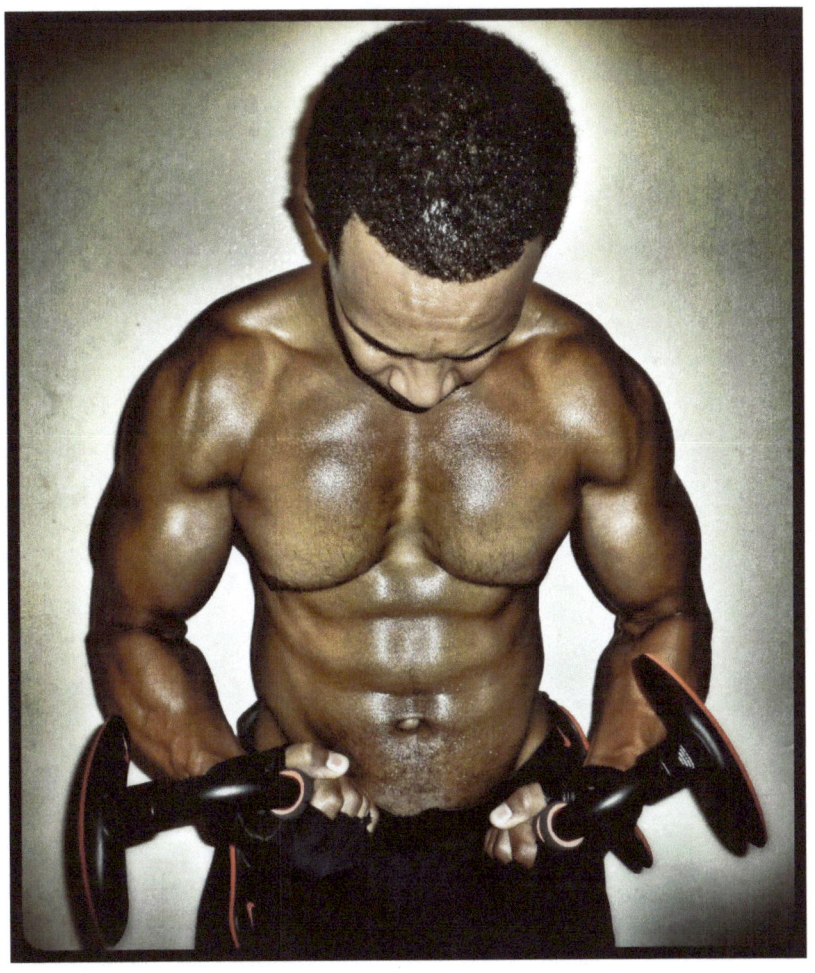

Chapter 1
LEVEL ONE
STANDARD STYLE

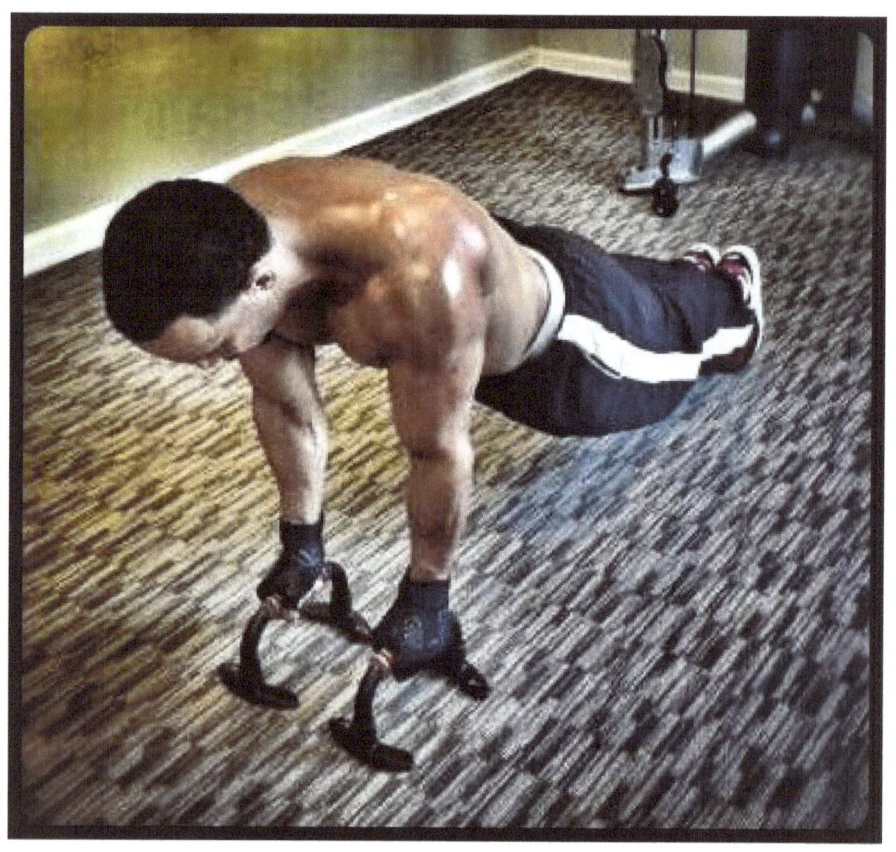

Variation #1
Regular Stance Push Up (Vertical/Close Feet)
Muscles Worked: Chest, Triceps, Abdominals, Shoulders

How to:

1. Place the push up bars about shoulder width apart in a vertical position. Grab both bars and elevate your upper body in the air. Fully extend your legs all the way out together with only your toes touching the floor. Keep your lower back and butt straight at all times. This is your starting position.

2. While breathing in, engage your core, then slowly lower your body straight down until your face is about 1-inch off the floor. Pause for a second at the bottom.

3. While breathing out, slowly raise your body back up to the starting position.

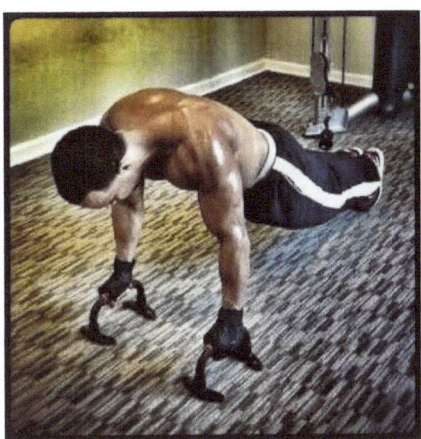 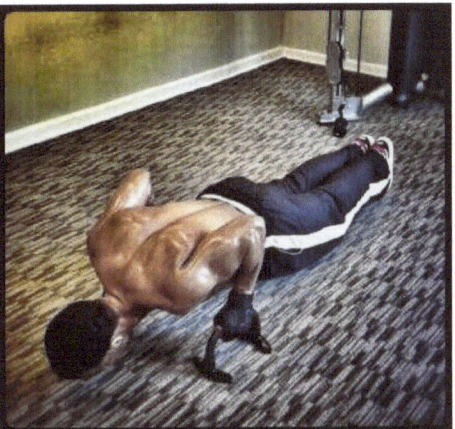

Variation #2

<u>Wide Stance Push Up</u> (Vertical/Close Feet)

Muscles Worked: Chest, Triceps, Abdominals, Shoulders

How to:

1. Place the push up bars about 6-inches past shoulder width apart on both sides in a vertical position. Grab both bars and elevate your upper body in the air. Fully extend your legs all the way out together with only your toes touching the floor. Keep your lower back and butt straight at all times. This is your starting position.

2. While breathing in, engage your core, then slowly lower your body straight down until your face is about 1-inch off the floor. Pause for a second at the bottom.

3. While breathing out, slowly raise your body back up to the starting position.

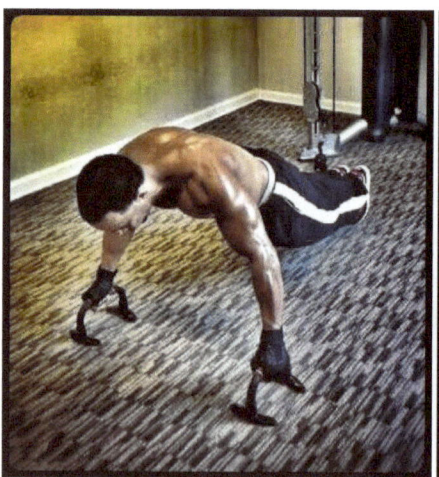 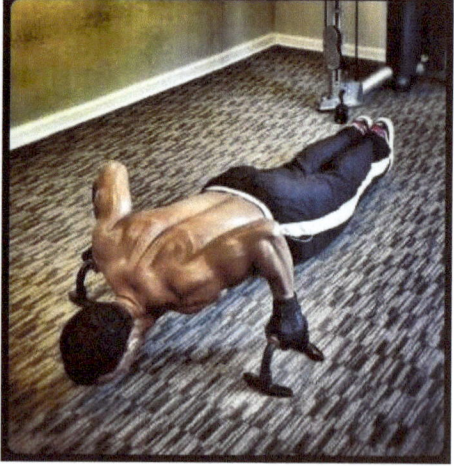

Variation #3

<u>Diamond Stance Push Up</u> (Diamond/Close Feet)
Muscles Worked: Chest, Triceps, Abdominals, Shoulders

How to:

1. Place the push up bars close together in the diamond-shaped position. Grab both bars and elevate your upper body in the air. Fully extend your legs all the way out together with only your toes touching the floor. Keep your lower back and butt straight at all times. This is your starting position.

2. While breathing in, engage your core, then slowly lower your body straight down until your face is about 1-inch off the floor. Pause for a second at the bottom.

3. While breathing out, slowly raise your body back up to the starting position.

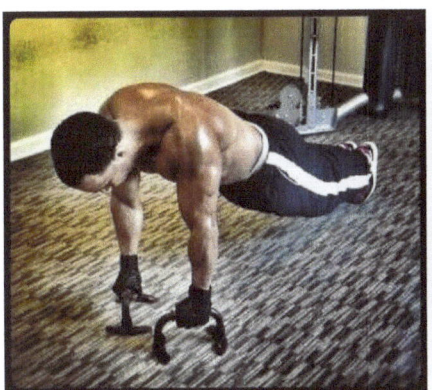 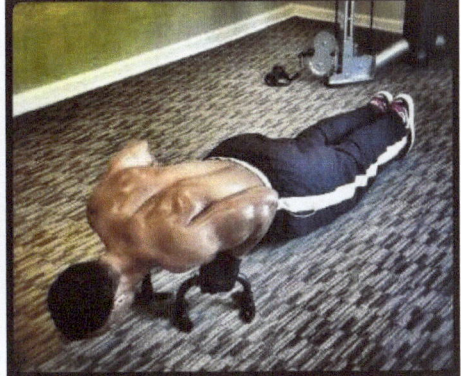

Variation #4

Hand On Bar/Hand On Floor Stance Push Up (Wide Feet)

Muscles Worked: Chest, Triceps, Abdominals, Shoulders

How to:

1. Place one push up bar about shoulder width apart in a horizontal position. Place your off hand with your palm faced down on the floor about shoulder width apart. Grab the one bar, and with the assistance of your off hand on the floor, elevate your upper body in the air. Fully extend your legs all the way out. Spread them wide as you can with only your toes touching the floor. Keep your lower back and butt straight at all times. This is your starting position.

2. While breathing in, engage your core, then slowly lower your body straight down until your face is about 1-inch off the floor. Pause for a second at the bottom. (Note: Because of the awkward position, maintain your balance at all times.)

3. While breathing out, slowly raise your body back up to the starting position. When set is completed, switch sides and repeat process.

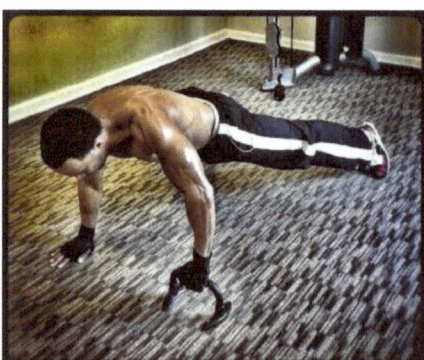 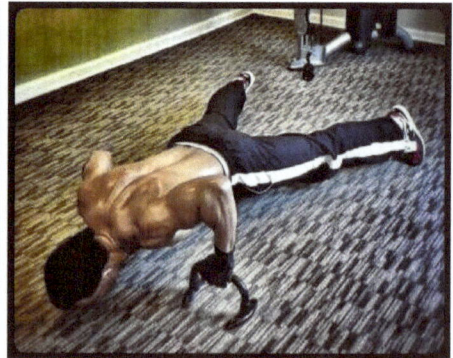

Variation #5

Close Stance Push Up (Vertical/Close Feet)
Muscles Worked: Chest, Triceps, Abdominals, Shoulders

How to:
1. Place the push up bars close together about 2-3 inches apart in a vertical position. Grab both bars and elevate your upper body in the air. Fully extend your legs all the way out together with only your toes touching the floor. Keep your lower back and butt straight at all times. This is your starting position.

2. While breathing in, engage your core, then slowly lower your body straight down until your face is about 1-inch off the floor. Pause for a second at the bottom.

3. While breathing out, slowly raise your body back up to the starting position.

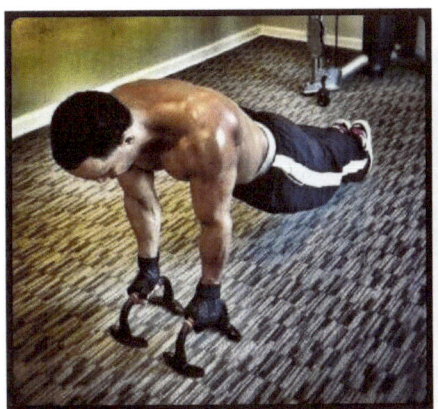 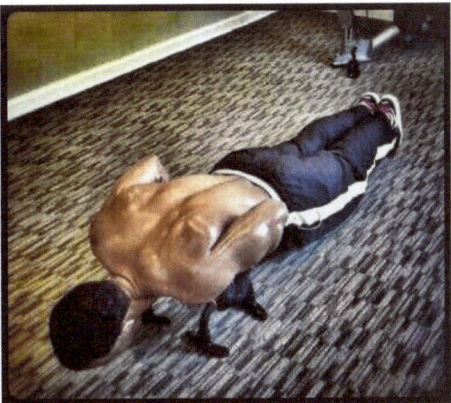

Variation #6

Hand On Bar/Knuckle On Floor Stance Push Up (Wide Feet)
Muscles Worked: Chest, Triceps, Abdominals, Shoulders

How to:

1. Place one push up bar about shoulder width apart in a vertical position. Place your off hand balled into a fist down on the floor about shoulder width apart. Grab the one bar, and with the assistance of your off hand (fist) on the floor, elevate your upper body in the air. Fully extend your legs all the way out. Spread them wide as you can with only your toes touching the floor. Keep your lower back and butt straight at all times. This is your starting position.

2. While breathing in, engage your core, then slowly lower your body straight down until your face 1-inch off the floor. Pause for a second at the bottom. (Note: Because of the awkward position, maintain your body at all times).

3. While breathing out, slowly raise your body back up to the starting position. When set is completed, switch sides and complete process.

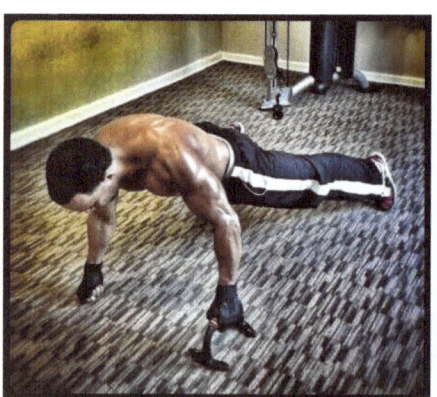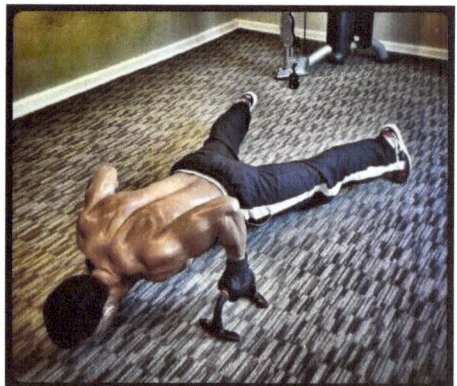

Variation #7

<u>Inverted Diamond Stance Push Up</u> (Inverted/Close Feet)
Muscles Worked: Chest, Triceps, Abdominals, Shoulders

How to:
1. Place the push up bars close together in the inverted or "backwards" diamond-shaped position. Grab both bars with an inverted grip and elevate your upper body in the air. Fully extend your legs all the way out together with only your toes touching the floor. Keep your lower back and butt straight at all times. This is your starting position.

2. While breathing in, engage your core, then slowly lower your body straight down until your face is about 1-inch off the floor. Pause for a second at the bottom.

3. While breathing out, slowly raise your body back up to the starting position.

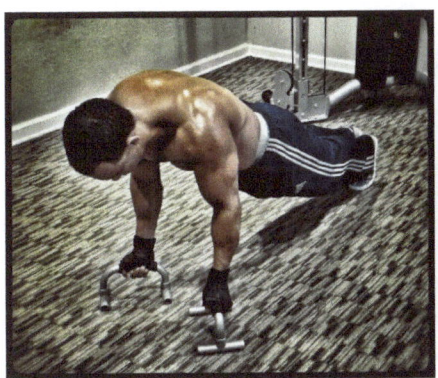 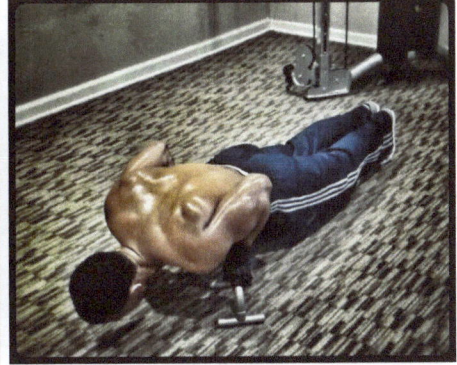

Variation #8

Reverse Bicep Stance Push Up (Horizontal/Close Feet)
Muscles Worked: Chest, Triceps, Abdominals, Shoulders

How to:

1. Place the push up bars about shoulder width apart in a horizontal position. Grab both bars with your wrists inverted, and elevate your upper body in the air. Fully extend your legs all the way out together with only your toes touching the floor. Keep your lower back and butt straight at all times. This is your starting position.

2. While breathing, engage your core, then slowly lower your body straight down until your face is about 1-inch off the floor. Pause for a second at the bottom.

3. While breathing out, slowly raise your body back up to the starting position.

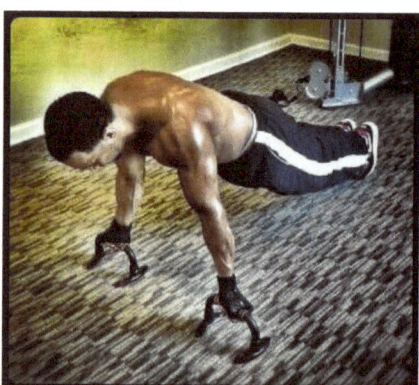 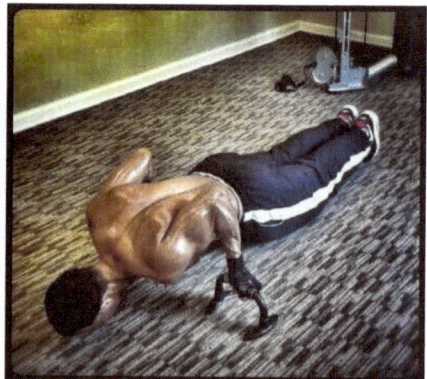

Chapter 2
LEVEL TWO
INTERMEDIATE STYLE

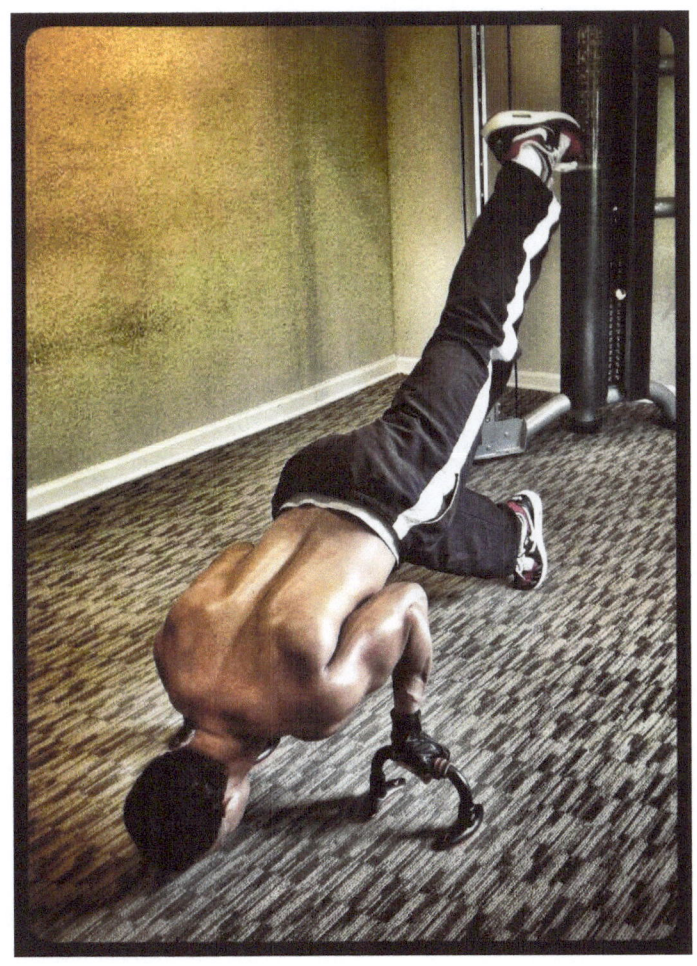

Variation #9

Elevated Leg Stance Push Up (Vertical)

Muscles Worked: Chest, Triceps, Abdominals, Shoulders, Legs

How to:

1. Place the push up bars about shoulder width apart in a vertical position. Grab both bars and elevate your upper body in the air. Fully extend your legs all the way out together with only your toes touching the floor. Then elevate your left leg up as high as you can with it fully extended and your toes pointed in the air. Keep your lower back and butt straight at all times. This is your starting position.

2. While breathing in, engage your core, then slowly lower your body straight down with your left leg continuing to stay elevated in the air until your face is about 1-inch off the floor. Pause for a second at the bottom.

3. While breathing out, slowly raise your body back up to the starting position. When set is completed, elevate right leg and repeat process.

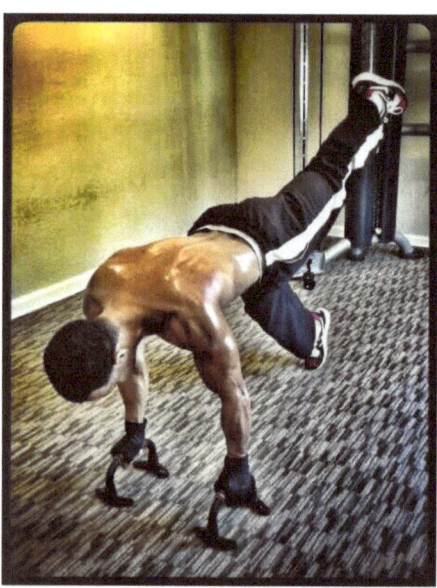 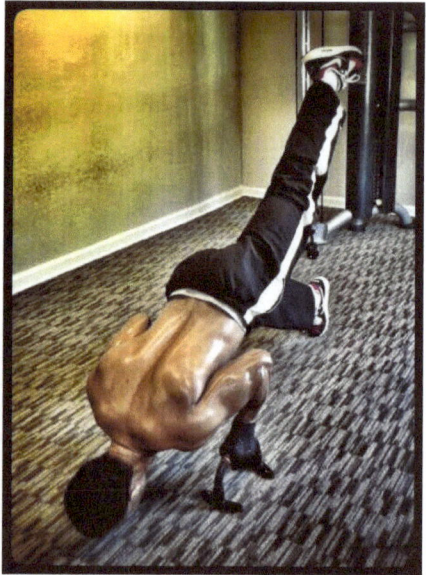

Variation #10
<u>High/Low Vertical Stance Push Up</u> (Wide Feet)
Muscles Worked: Chest, Triceps, Abdominals, Shoulders

How to:
1. Place the push up bars about 2-inches beyond shoulder width apart in a High/Low vertical position. The right bar should be positioned slightly in front of your head area, and the left bar should be positioned just parallel to your chest area. Grab both bars and elevate your upper body in the air. Fully extend your legs all the way out. Spread them as wide as you can with only your toes touching the floor. Keep your lower back and butt straight at all times. This is your starting position.

2. While breathing in, engage your core, then slowly your body straight down until your face is about 1-inch off the floor. Pause for a second at the bottom.

3. While breathing out, slowly raise your body back up to the starting position. When set is completed, switch the bar sides and repeat process.

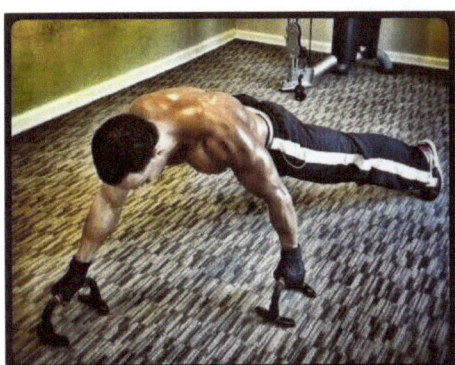 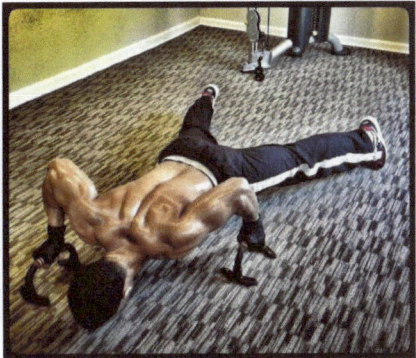

Variation #11
<u>Vertical Bar/Horizontal Bar Stance Push Up</u> (Wide Feet)
Muscles Worked: Chest, Triceps, Abdominals, Shoulders

How to:
1. Place the push up bars about shoulder width apart. The left side in the vertical position, and the right side in the horizontal position. Grab both bars and elevate your upper body in the air. Fully extend your legs all the way out. Spread them as wide as you can with only your toes touching the floor. Keep your lower back and butt straight at all times. This is your starting position.

2. While breathing in, engage your core, then slowly lower your body straight down until your face is about 1-inch off the floor. Pause for one second at the bottom.

3. While breathing out, slowly raise your body back up to the starting position. When set is completed, switch the bar sides and repeat process.

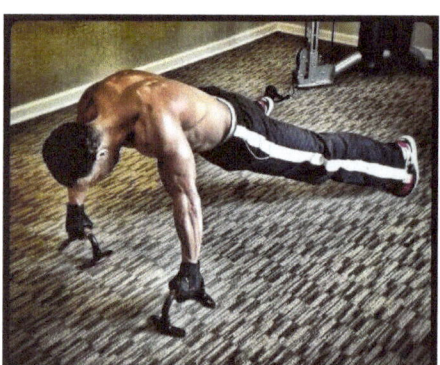 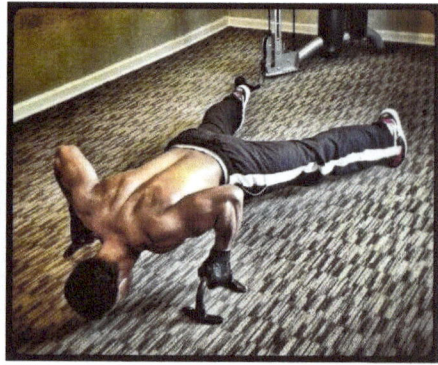

Variation #12

Diamond Elevated Leg Stance Push Up (Diamond)
Muscles Worked: Chest, Triceps, Abdominals, Shoulders, Legs

How to:

1. Place the push up bars close together in the diamond-shaped position. Grab both bars and elevate your upper body in the air. Fully extend your legs all the way out together with only your toes touching the floor. Then elevate your left leg up as high as you can with it fully extended and your toes pointed in the air. Keep your lower back and butt straight at all times. This is your starting position.

2. While breathing in, engage your core, then slowly lower your body straight down with your left leg continuing to stay elevated in the air until your face is about 1-inch off the floor. Pause for a second at the bottom.

3. While breathing out, slowly raise your body back up to the starting position. When set is completed, elevate right leg and repeat process.

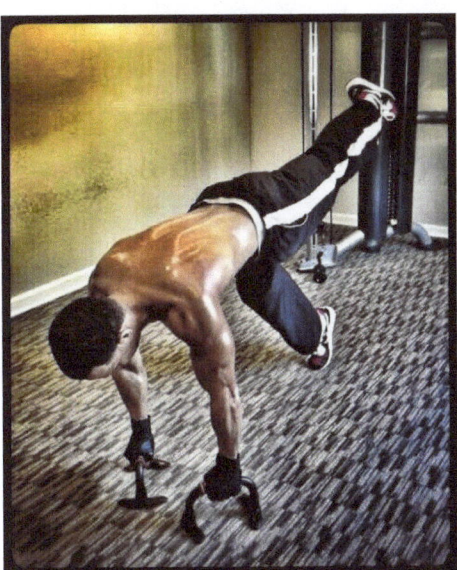 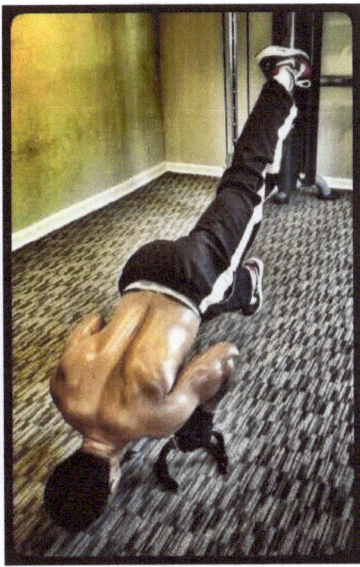

Variation #13

Decline Elevated Feet Stance Push Up/On-Bench (Vertical/Close Feet)
Muscles Worked: Chest, Triceps, Abdominals, Shoulders, Legs

How to:

1. Place the push up bars about shoulder width apart in a vertical position. Grab both bars and elevate your upper body in the air while placing both feet on the bench together. Make sure your body is fully extended and your lower back and butt are straight at all times. This is your starting position.

2. While breathing in, engage your core, then slowly lower your body straight down until your face is about 1-inch off the floor. Your body should be in the decline position at this point. Pause for a second at the bottom.

3. While breathing out, slowly raise your body back up to the starting position.

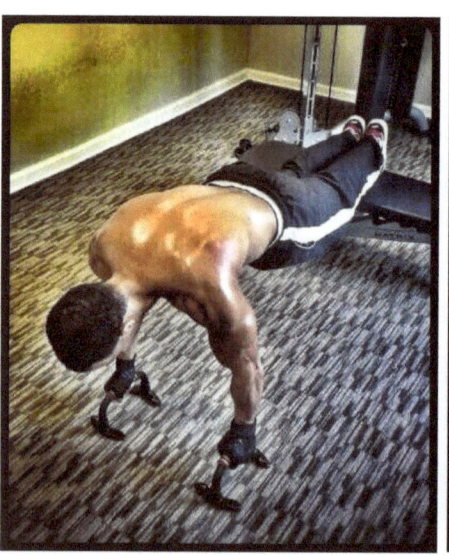 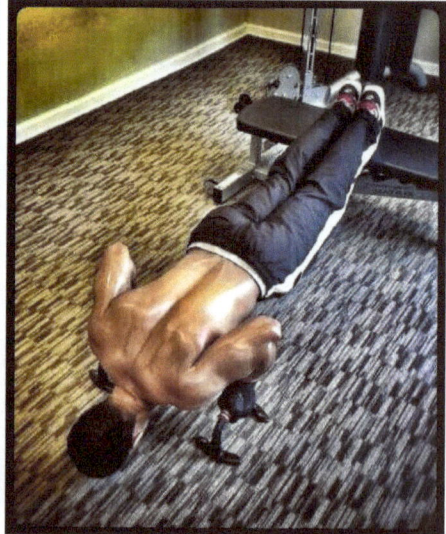

Variation #14

Decline Diamond Elevated Feet Stance Push Up/On-Bench (Diamond/Close Feet)
Muscles Worked: Chest, Triceps, Abdominals, Shoulders, Legs

How to:
1. Place the push up bars close together in the diamond-shaped position. Grab both bars and elevate your upper body in the air while placing both feet on the bench together. Make sure your body is fully extended and your lower back and butt are straight at all times. This is your starting position.

2. While breathing in, engage your core, then slowly lower your body straight down until your face is about 1-inch off the floor. Your body should be in the decline position at this point. Pause for a second at the bottom.

3. While breathing out, slowly raise your body back up to the starting position.

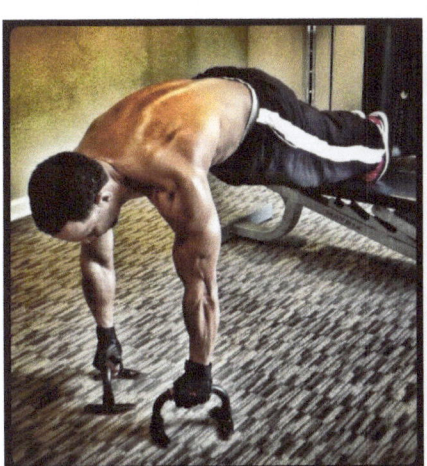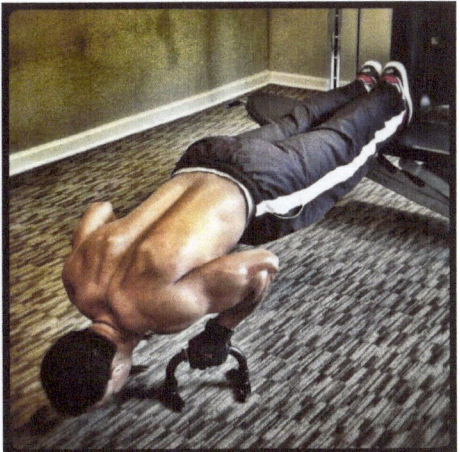

Variation #15

<u>Reverse Bicep Elevated Leg Stance Push Up</u> (Horizontal)
Muscles Worked: Chest, Triceps, Abdominals, Shoulders, Legs

How to:

1. Place the push up bars about shoulder width apart in a horizontal position. Grab both bars with your wrists inverted and elevate your upper body in the air. Fully extend your legs all the way out together with only your toes touching the floor. Then elevate your left leg up as high as you can with it fully extended and your toes pointed in the air. Keep your lower back and butt straight at all times. This is your starting position.

2. While breathing in, engage your core, then slowly lower your body straight down with your left leg continuing to stay elevated in the air until your face is about 1-inch off the floor. Pause for a second at the bottom.

3. While breathing out, slowly raise your body back up to the starting position. When set is completed, elevate right leg and repeat process.

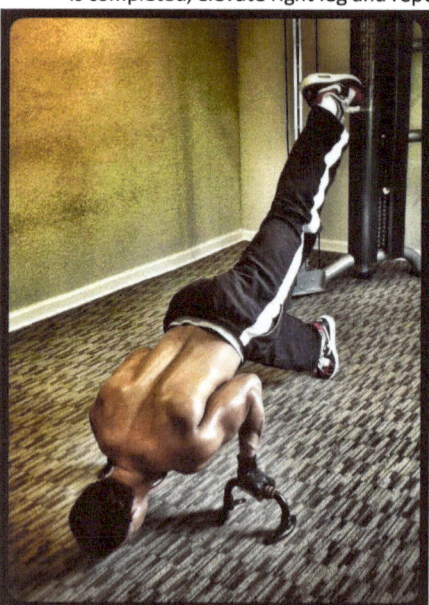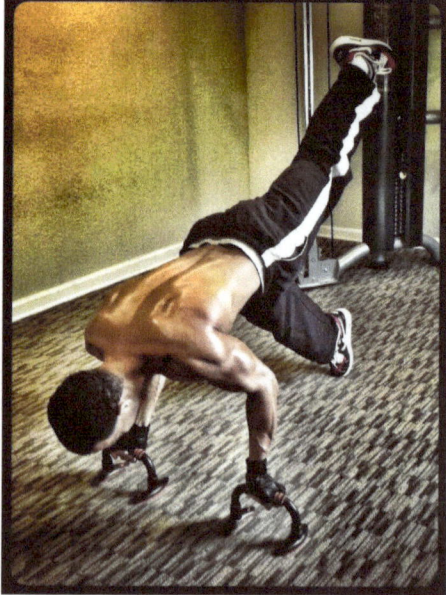

Variation #16

<u>Decline Reverse Bicep Elevated Feet Stance Push Up/On-Bench</u> (Close Feet)
Muscles Worked: Chest, Triceps, Abdominals, Shoulders, Legs

How to:
1. Place the push up bars about shoulder width apart in a horizontal position. Grab both bars with your wrists inverted and elevate your upper body in the air while placing both feet on the bench together. Make sure your body is fully extended and your lower back and butt are straight at all times. This is your starting position.

2. While breathing in, engage your core, then slowly lower your body straight down until your face is about 1-inch off the floor. Your body should be in the decline position at this point. Pause for a second at the bottom.

3. While breathing out, slowly raise your body back up to the starting position.

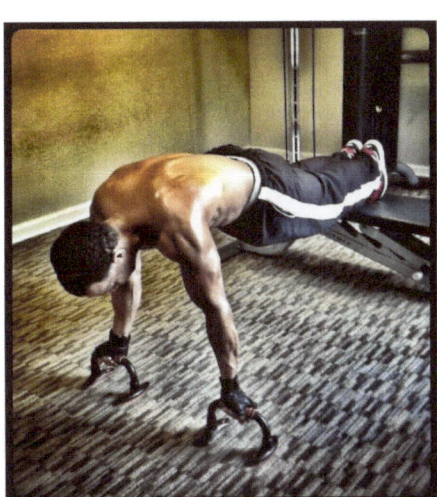 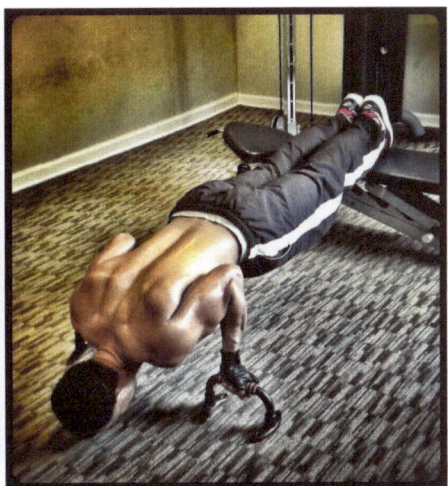

Variation #17

Inverted Diamond Elevated Leg Stance Push Up (Inverted)

Muscles Worked: Chest, Triceps, Abdominals, Shoulders, Legs

How to:

1. Place the push up bars close together in the inverted or "backwards" diamond-shaped position. Grab both bars with an inverted grip and elevate your upper body in the air. Fully extend your legs all the way out together with only your toes touching the floor. Then elevate your left leg up as high as you can with it fully extended and your toes pointed in the air. Keep your lower back and butt straight at all times. This is your starting position.

2. While breathing in, engage your core, then slowly lower your body straight down with your left leg continuing to stay elevated in the air until your face is about 1-inch off the floor. Pause for a second at the bottom.

3. While breathing out, slowly raise your body back up to the starting position. When set is completed, elevate right leg and repeat process.

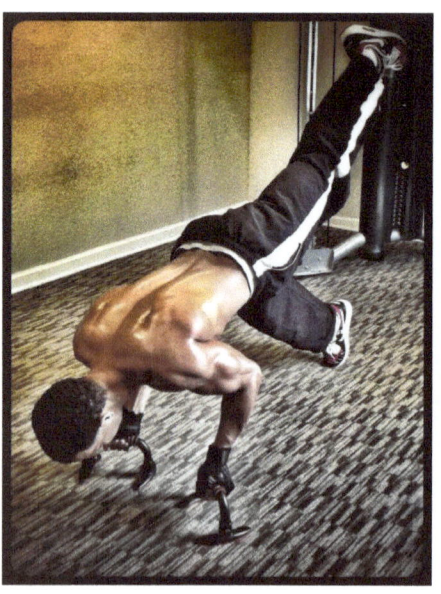 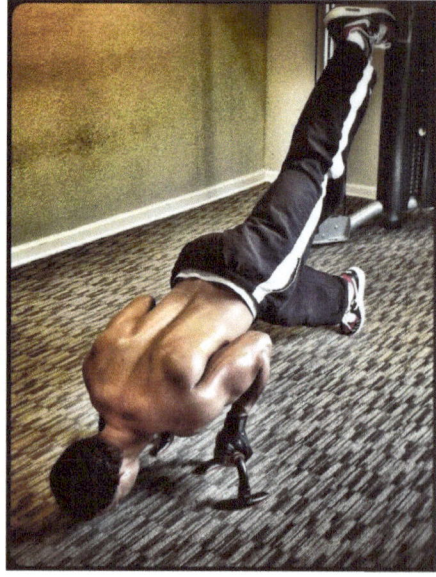

Variation #18

Decline Inverted Diamond Elevated Feet Stance Push Up/On-Bench (Close Feet)
Muscles Worked: Chest, Triceps, Abdominals, Shoulders, Legs

How to:
1. Place the push up bars close together in the inverted or "backwards" diamond-shaped position. Grab both bars with an inverted grip and elevate your upper body in the air while placing both feet on the bench together. Make sure your body is fully extended and your lower back and butt are straight at all times. This is your starting position.

2. While breathing in, engage your core, then slowly lower your body straight down until your face is about 1-inch off the floor. Your body should be in the decline position at this point. Pause for a second at the bottom.

3. While breathing out, slowly raise your body back up to the starting position.

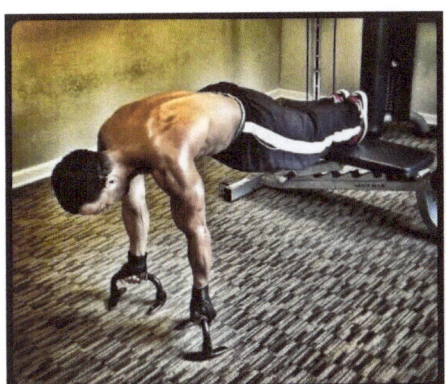 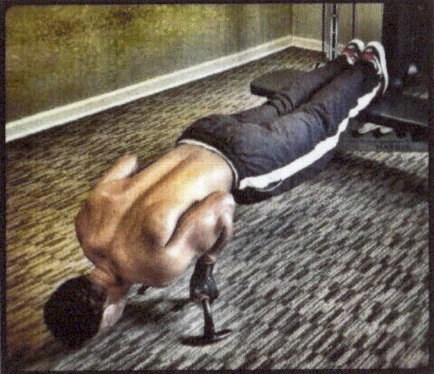

Variation #19

<u>Overhand/Underhand High/Low Stance Push Up</u> (Wide Feet)
Muscles Worked: Chest, Triceps, Abdominals, Shoulders

How to:
1. Place the push up bars about 2-inches beyond shoulder width apart in a High/Low horizontal position. The right bar should be positioned slightly in front of your head area, and the left bar should be positioned just parallel to your chest area. Grab both bars with your right hand using an overhand grip, and your left hand using an underhand grip; then elevate your upper body in the air. Fully extend your legs all the way out. Spread them as wide as you can with only your toes touching the floor. Keep your lower back and butt straight at all times. This is your starting position.

2. While breathing in, engage your core, then slowly lower your body straight down until your face is about 1-inch off the floor. Pause for a second at the bottom.

3. While breathing out, slowly raise your body back up to the starting position. When set is completed, switch the bar sides and repeat process.

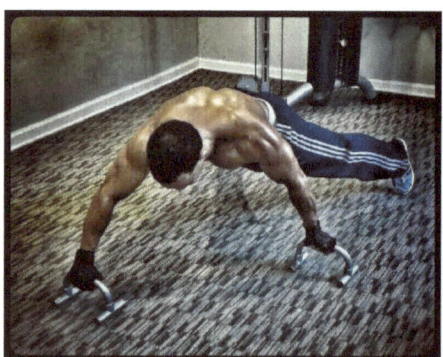 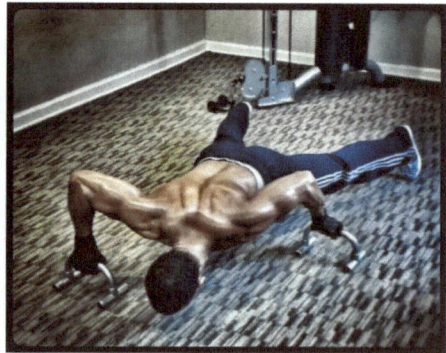

Variation #20
<u>Walk Side-to-Side Stance Push Up</u> (Vertical/Close Feet)
Muscles Worked: Chest, Triceps, Abdominals, Shoulders

How to:
1. Place the push up bars about shoulder width apart in a vertical position. Grab both bars and elevate your upper body in the air. Fully extend your legs all the way out together with only your toes touching the floor. Keep your lower back and butt straight at all times. This is your starting position.

2. While breathing in and out, engage your core, then remove your left hand off the left bar and place it in the center of the floor in between the two push up bars with your palm faced down. Keep your right hand on the right bar, then complete a push up by slowly lowering your body straight down until your face is about 1-inch off the floor. Pause for a second at the bottom, then in reverse repeat the process for the right side.

3. When set is completed, return back to the starting position.

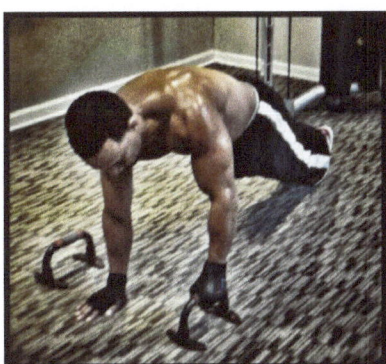 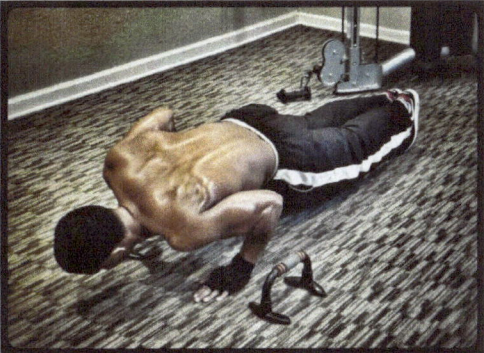

Variation #21

Typewriter Stance Push Up (Vertical/Wide Feet)
Muscles Worked: Chest, Triceps, Abdominals, Shoulders

How to:

1. Place the push up bars full arm length apart and in vertical position. Grab both bars and elevate your upper body in the air. Fully extend your legs all the way out. Spread them as wide as you can with only your toes touching the floor. Keep your lower back and butt straight at all times. This is your starting position.

2. While breathing in and out, engage your core, then slowly shift your body downward all the way to the right until your left arm is fully extended horizontally from the left push up bar. Pause for a second, then rotate your body all the way to the left until your right arm is fully extended horizontally from the right push up bar. Pause for a second.

3. When left and right side reps are completed, raise your body back up to the starting position.

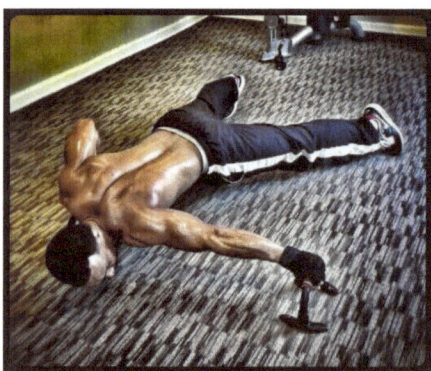 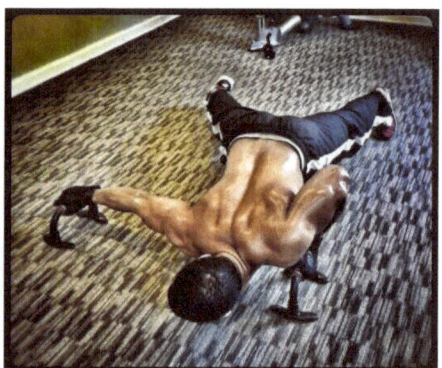

Variation #22
Grasshopper Stance Push Up (Vertical/Close Feet)
Muscles Worked: Chest, Triceps, Abdominals, Shoulders, Legs

How to:
1. Place the push up bars about shoulder width apart in a vertical position. Grab both bars and elevate your upper body in the air. Fully extend your legs all the way out together with only your toes touching the floor. Keep your lower back and butt straight at all times. This is your starting position.

2. While breathing in, engage your core, then slowly lower your body down while rotating your hips until your right knee is vertical to the left push up bar. Pause for a second at the bottom.

3. While breathing out, slowly rotate your body back up to the starting position and repeat process for the right side.

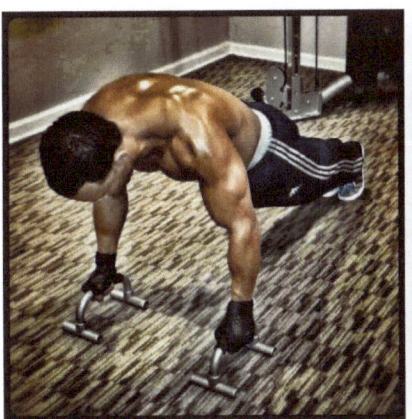 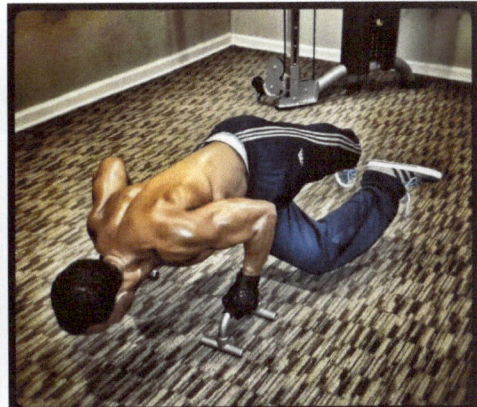

Chapter 3
LEVEL THREE
ADVANCED STYLE

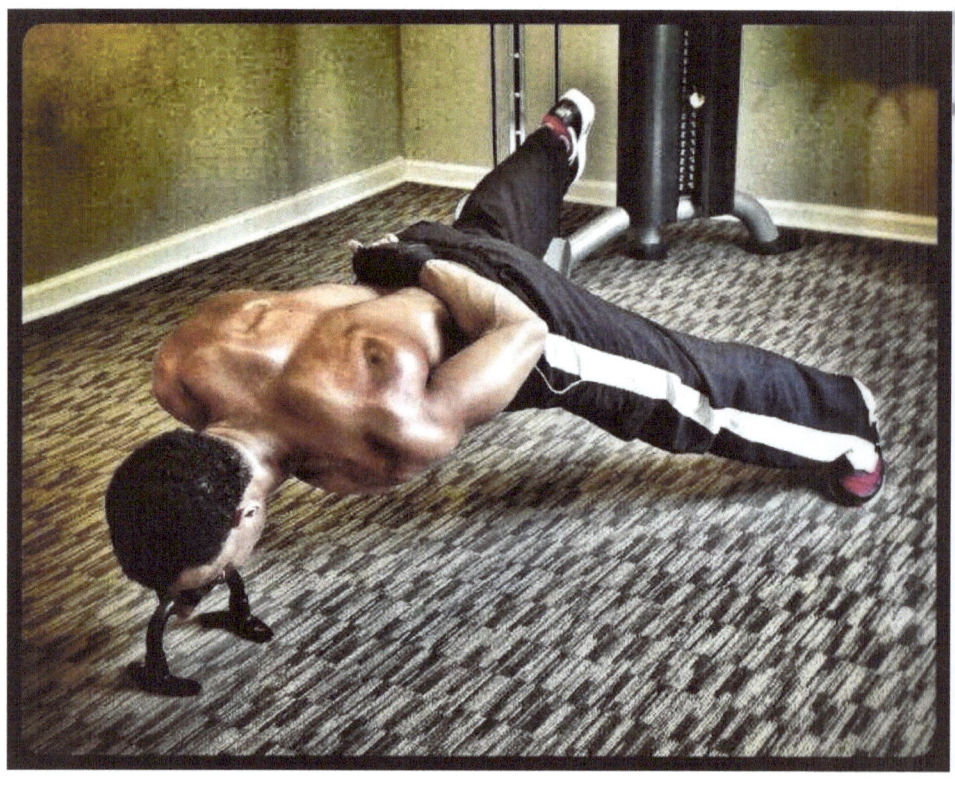

Variation #23
Balance Beam Stance Push Up (Horizontal/Close Feet)
Muscles Worked: Chest, Triceps, Abdominals, Shoulders

How to:
1. Place the push up bars about body length apart in a horizontal position. Carefully climb on top of each push up bar by placing the tips of your toes on top of the bar behind you, and gripping the bar in front of you with a two-hand grip. Elevate your body all the way up until your arms are fully extended up. Keep your lower back and butt straight at all times. This is your starting position.

2. While breathing in, engage your core, then slowly lower your body straight down until your face is about 4-6 inches off the floor. Pause for a second at the bottom. *Note: Maintain extreme balance and caution at all times when attempting this exercise.*

3. While breathing out, slowly raise your body back up to the starting position.

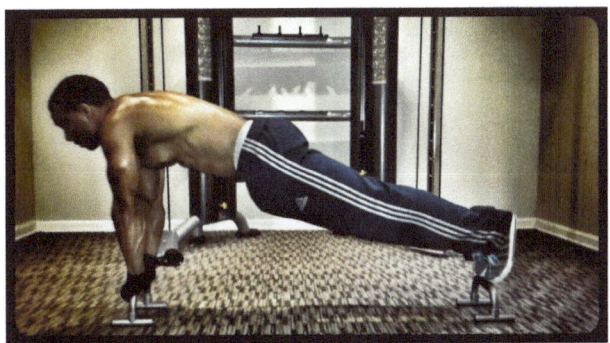

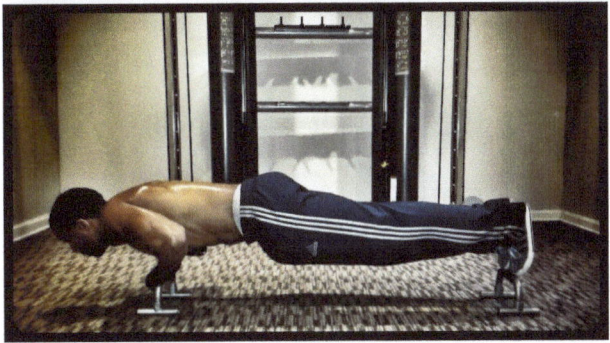

Variation #24

Balance Beam Elevated Leg Stance Push Up (Horizontal)
Muscles Worked: Chest, Triceps, Abdominals, Shoulders, Legs

How to:

1. Place the push up bars about body length apart in a horizontal position. Carefully climb on top of each push up bar by placing the tips of your toes on top of the bar behind, and gripping the bar in front of you with a two-hand grip. Elevate your body all the way up until your arms are fully extended up. Then elevate your left leg up as high as you can with it fully extended and your toes pointed in the air. Keep your lower back and butt straight at all times. This is your starting position.

2. While breathing in, engage your core, then slowly lower your body straight down with your left leg continuing to stay elevated in the air until your face is about 4-6 inches off the floor. Pause for a second at the bottom. *Note: Maintain extreme balance and caution at all times when attempting this exercise.*

3. While breathing out, slowly raise your body back up to the starting position. When set is completed, elevate right leg and repeat process.

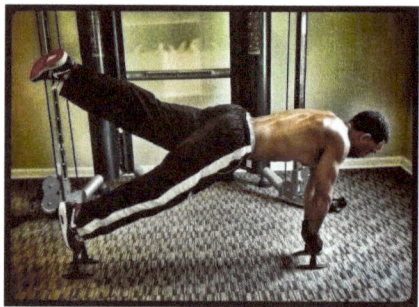 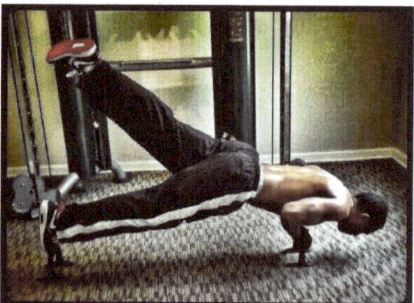

Variation #25
Tucked Planche Stance Push Up (Vertical)
Muscles Worked: Chest, Triceps, Abdominals, Shoulders, Legs

How to:

1. Place the push up bars about 2-inches beyond shoulder width apart in a vertical position. Grab both bars, then elevate your body up in the air with your knees tucked up towards your chest area with your arms fully extended out. Your legs/feet should be about 4-6 inches off the floor. This is your starting position.

2. While breathing in, engage your core, then slowly lower your body straight down while maintaining the tuck position until your legs/feet are about 1-2 inches off the floor. Pause for a second at the bottom.

3. While breathing out, slowly raise your body back up to the starting position.

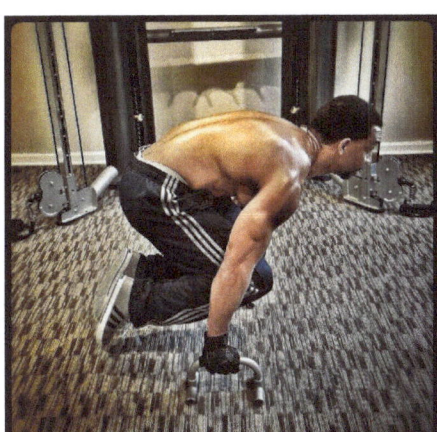 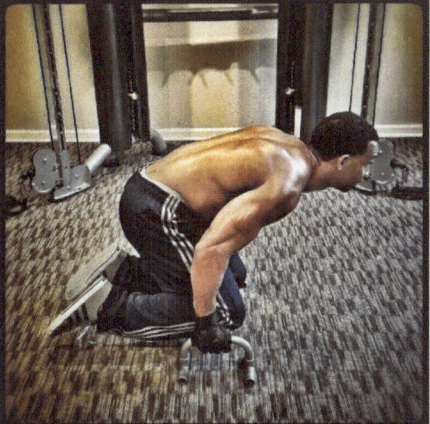

Variation #26
Decline Elevated Leg Off-Bench Stance Push Up (Vertical)
Muscles Worked: Chest, Triceps, Abdominals, Shoulders, Legs

How to:
1. Place the push up bars about shoulder width apart in a vertical position. Grab both bars and elevate your upper body in the air while placing both feet on the bench together. Then elevate your left leg up as high as you can with it fully extended and your toes pointed in the air. Make sure your body is fully extended and your lower back and butt are straight at all times. This is your starting position.

2. While breathing in, engage your core, then slowly lower your body straight down with your left leg continuing to stay elevated in the air until your face is about 1-inch off the floor. Your body should be in the decline position at this point. Pause for a second at the bottom.

3. While breathing out, slowly raise your body back up to the starting position. When set is completed, elevate right leg and repeat process.

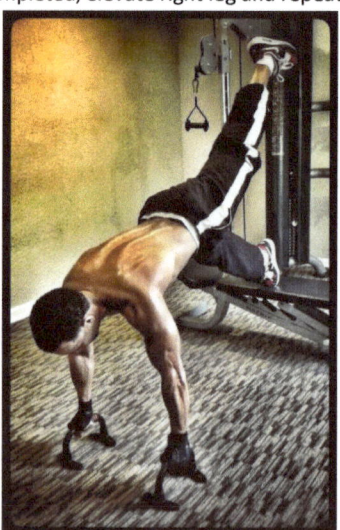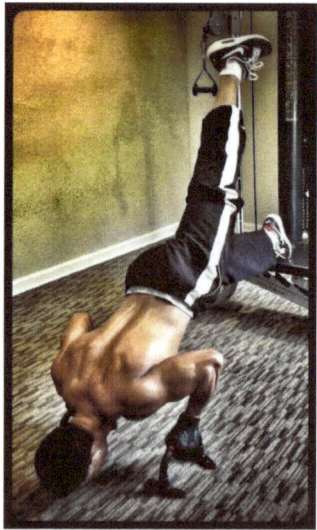

Variation #27
<u>Decline Diamond Elevated Leg Off-Bench Stance Push Up</u> (Diamond)
Muscles Worked: Chest, Triceps, Abdominals, Shoulders, Legs

How to:
1. Place the push up bars close together in the diamond-shaped position. Grab both bars and elevate your upper body in the air while placing both feet on the bench together. Then elevate your left leg up as high as you can with it fully extended and your toes pointed in the air. Make sure your body is fully extended and your lower back and butt are straight at all times. This is your starting position.

2. While breathing in, engage your core, then slowly lower your body straight down with your left leg continuing to stay elevated in the air until your face is about 1-inch off the floor. Your body should be in the decline position at this point. Pause for a second at the bottom.

3. While breathing out, slowly raise your body back up to the starting position. When set is completed, elevate right leg and repeat process.

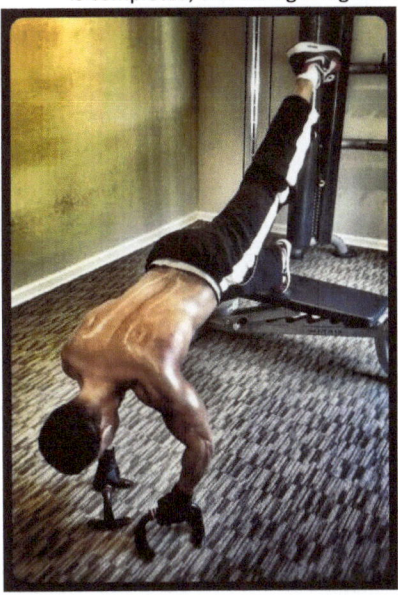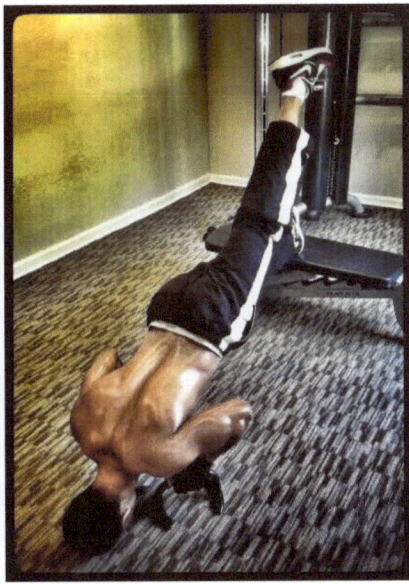

Variation #28

Decline Inverted Diamond Elevated Leg Off-Bench Stance Push Up (Inverted)
Muscles Worked: Chest, Triceps, Abdominals, Shoulders, Legs

How to:

1. Place the push up bars close together in the inverted or "backwards" diamond-shaped position. Grab both bars with an inverted grip and elevate your upper body in the air while placing both feet on the bench together. Then elevate your left leg up as high as you can with it fully extended and your toes pointed in the air. Make sure your body is fully extended and your lower back and butt are straight at all times. This is your starting position.

2. While breathing in, engage your core, then slowly lower your body straight down with your left leg continuing to stay elevated in the air until your face is about 1-inch off the floor. Your body should be in the decline position at this point. Pause for a second at the bottom.

3. While breathing out, slowly raise your body back up to the starting position. When set is completed, elevate right leg and repeat process.

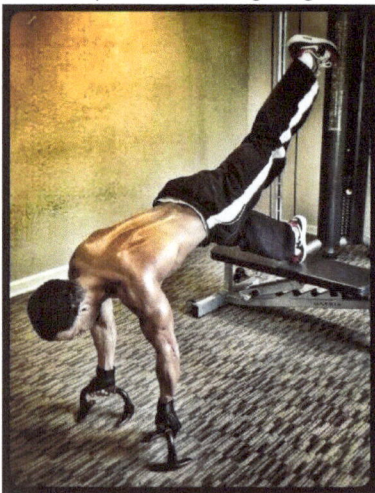 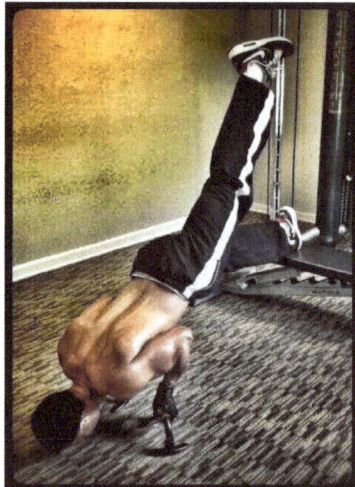

Variation #29
Decline Reverse Bicep Elevated Leg Off-Bench Stance Push Up (Horizontal)
Muscles Worked: Chest, Triceps, Abdominals, Shoulders, Legs

How to:
1. Place the push up bars about shoulder width apart in a horizontal position. Grab both bars with your wrists inverted and elevate your upper body in the air while placing both feet on the bench together. Then elevate your left leg up as high as you can with it fully extended and your toes pointed in the air. Make sure your body is fully extended and your lower back and butt are straight at all times. This is your starting position.

2. While breathing in, engage your core, then slowly lower your body straight down with your left leg continuing to stay elevated in the air until your face is about 1-inch off the floor. Your body should be in the decline position at this point. Pause for a second at the bottom.

3. While breathing out, slowly raise your body back up to the starting position. When set is completed, elevate right leg and repeat process.

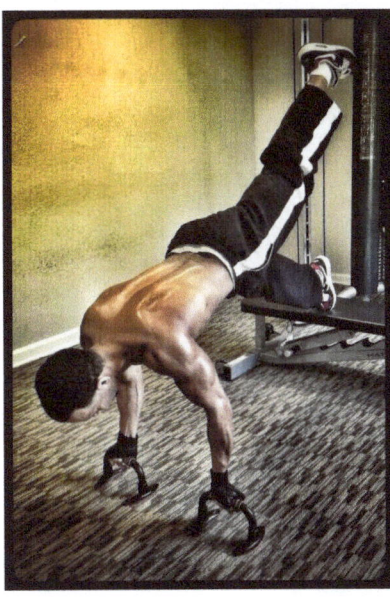 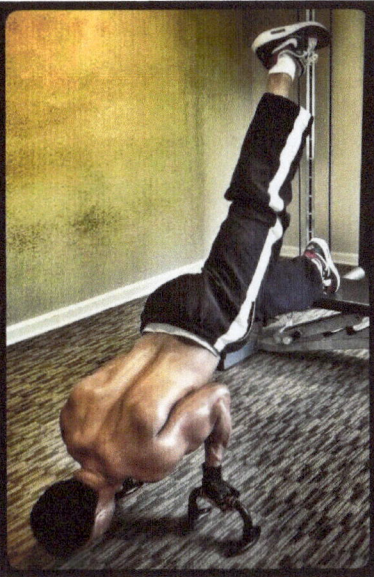

Variation #30

<u>Extra Wide Diamond Stance Push Up</u> (Wide Feet)
Muscles Worked: Chest, Triceps, Abdominals, Shoulders

How to:

1. Place the push up bars about 6-8 inches past shoulder width apart on both sides in the diamond-shaped position. Grab both bars and elevate your upper body in the air. Fully extend your legs all the way out. Spread them as wide as you can with only your toes touching the floor. Keep your lower back and butt straight at all times. This is your starting position.

2. While breathing in, engage your core, then slowly lower your body straight down until your face is about 1-inch off the floor. Pause for a second at the bottom. *Note: Because of the awkward position, maintain your balance at all times.*

3. While breathing out, slowly raise your body back up to the starting position.

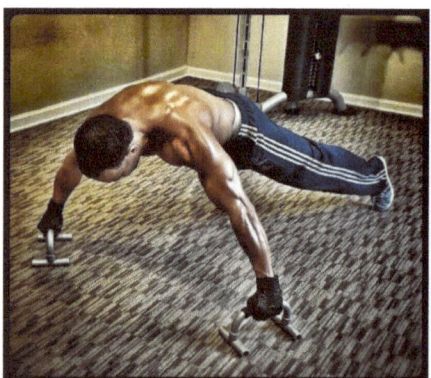 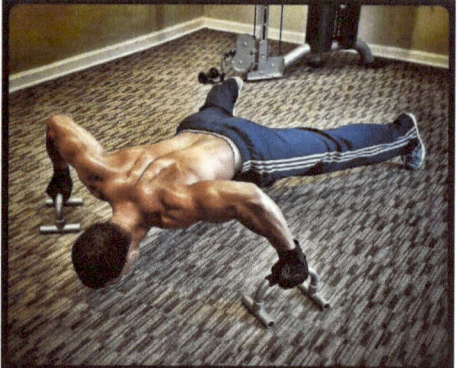

Variation #31

<u>Extra Wide Inverted Diamond Stance Push Up</u> (Wide Feet)
Muscles Worked: Chest, Triceps, Abdominals, Shoulders

How to:
1. Place the push up bars about 6-8 inches past shoulder width apart on both sides in the inverted or "backwards" diamond-shaped position. Grab both bars with an inverted grip and elevate your upper body in the air. Fully extend your legs all the way out. Spread them as wide as you can with only your toes touching the floor. Keep your lower back and butt straight at all times. This is your starting position.

2. While breathing in, engage your core, then slowly lower your body straight down until your face is about 1-inch off the floor. Pause for a second at the bottom. *Note: Because of the awkward position, maintain your balance at all times.*

3. While breathing out, slowly raise your body back up to the starting position.

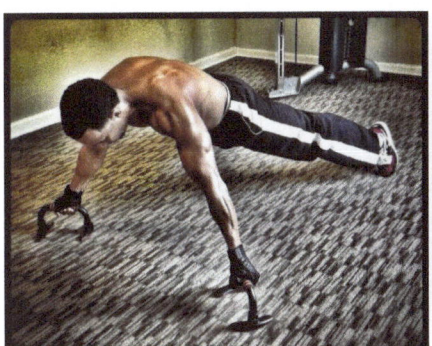 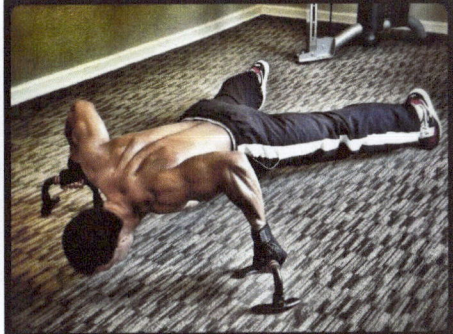

Variation #32

Single Bar Two Hand Grip Stance Push Up (Close Feet/Vertical)
Muscles Worked: Chest, Triceps, Abdominals, Shoulders

How to:

1. Place 1 single push up bar on the floor parallel to your chest region in a vertical position. Grab the bar with an overhand/underhand grip and elevate your upper body in the air. Fully extend your legs all the way out together with only your toes touching the floor. Keep your lower back and butt straight at all times. This is your starting position.

2. While breathing in, engage your core, then slowly lower your body straight down until your face is about 1-inch off the floor. Pause for a second at the bottom: *Note: Because of the awkward position, maintain your balance at all times.*

3. While breathing out, slowly raise your body back up to the starting position.

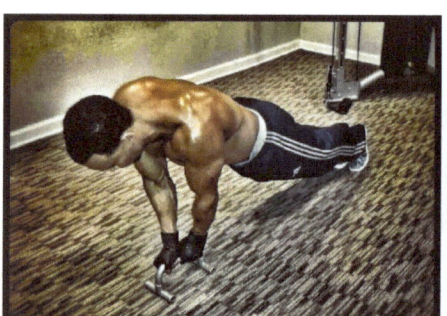 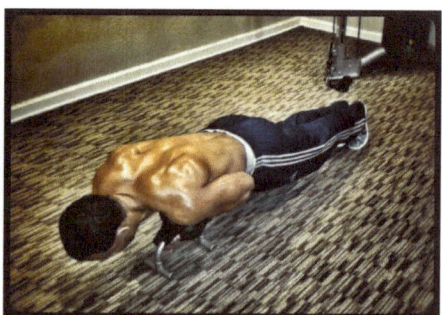

Variation #33
Tricep Nose Dive Stance Push Up (Horizontal/Close Feet)
Muscles Worked: Chest, Triceps, Abdominals, Shoulders

How to:
1. Place the push up bars close together in a horizontal position. Grab both bars with an overhand false grip with your thumbs placed on top of the push up bars. Then elevate your upper body in the air. Fully extend your legs all the way out together with only your toes touching the floor. Keep your lower back and butt straight at all times. This is your starting position.

2. While breathing in, engage your core, then slowly lower your body straight down until your elbows are about 1-inch off the floor. Pause for a second at the bottom. *Note: Your triceps must be very strong to complete this exercise.*

3. While breathing out, slowly raise your body back up to the starting position.

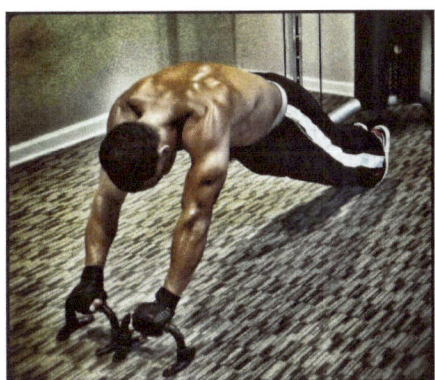 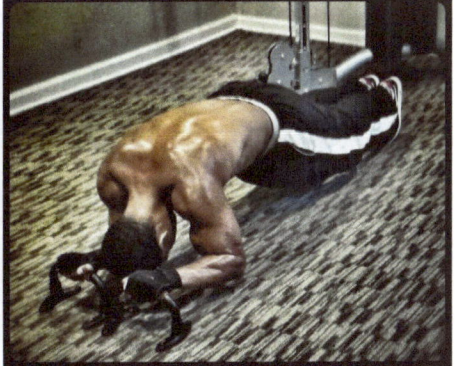

Variation #34

Elevated Head Stand Shoulder Stance Push Up (Vertical/Close Feet)
Muscles Worked: Chest, Triceps, Abdominals, Shoulders, Legs

How to:

1. Place the push up bars about 6-8 inches away from the bench approximately shoulder width apart in a vertical position. Grab both bars and place your feet on the bench. Raise your feet up until you are on the balls of your feet. Elevate your butt up as high as possible and position the crown of your head in the air between the push up bars. Make sure your wrists and butt are in alignment with each other. This is your starting position.

2. While breathing in, engage your core, then slowly lower your body straight down until the crown of your head taps the floor. Your body should be in an upside down L-shape position at this point. Pause for a second at the bottom. *Note: Because of the awkward position, maintain your balance at all times.*

3. While breathing out, slowly raise your body back up to the starting position.

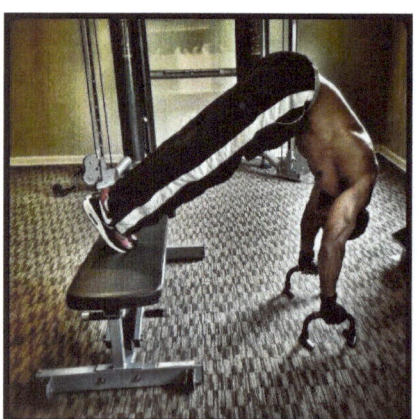 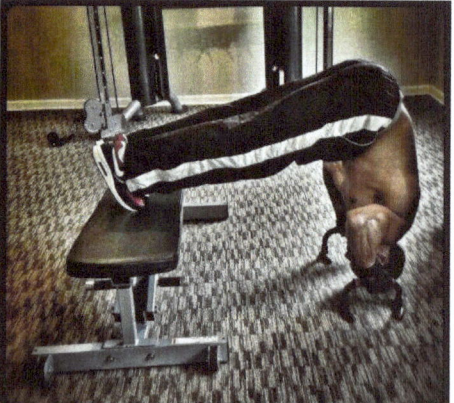

Variation #35

<u>One-Arm/One-Bar Wide Stance Push Up</u> (Vertical/Wide Feet)

Muscles Worked: Chest, Triceps, Abdominals, Shoulders

How to:

1. Place 1 single push up bar in alignment with your right shoulder in a vertical position. Grab the one bar with your right hand and elevate your upper body in the air with your right arm fully extended up. Place your left hand behind your back and fully extend your legs all the way out. Spread them as wide as you can with only your toes touching the floor. Keep your lower back and butt straight at all times. This is your starting position.

2. While breathing in, engage your core, then slowly lower your body straight down until your face is about 1-2 inches off the floor. Pause for a second at the bottom. *Note: Because of the awkward position, maintain your balance at all times.*

3. While breathing out, slowly raise your body back up to the starting position. When set is completed, switch exercise to left arm and repeat process.

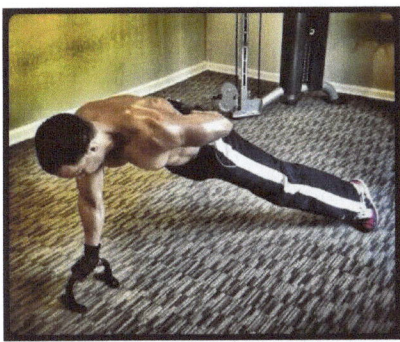 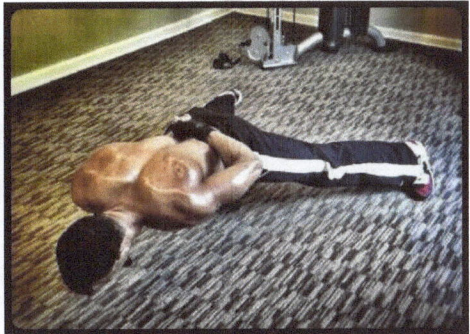

Variation #36

One-Arm/One-Bar/One-Leg Wide Stance Push Up (Vertical/Wide Feet)
Muscles Worked: Chest, Triceps, Abdominals, Shoulders, Legs

How to:

1. Place one single push up bar in alignment with your right shoulder in a vertical position. Grab the one bar with your right hand and elevate your upper body in the air with your right arm fully extended up. Place your left hand behind your back and fully extend your legs all the way out. Spread them as wide as you can with only your toes touching the floor. Then elevate your right leg off the floor about 4-6 inches. Keep your lower back and butt straight at all times. This is your starting position.

2. While breathing in, engage your core, then slowly lower your body straight down until your face is about 1-2 inches off the floor. Pause for a second at the bottom. *Note: Because of the awkward position, maintain your balance at all times.*

3. While breathing out, slowly raise your body back up to the starting position. When set is completed, switch exercise to left arm, then elevate your left leg and repeat process.

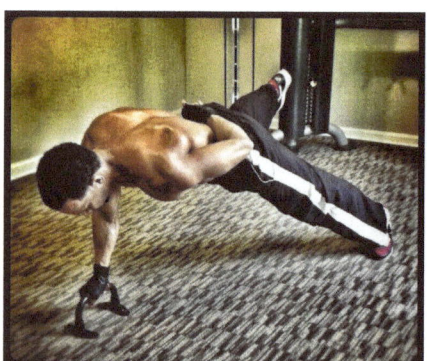 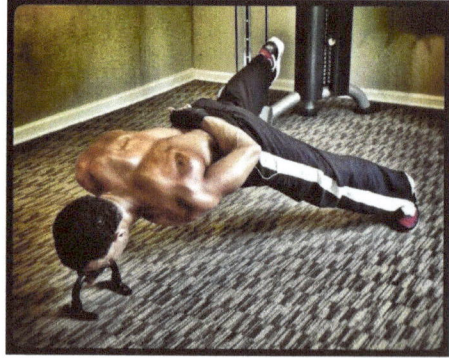

Variation #37

Decline One-Arm/One-Bar/Elevated Feet On Bench Wide Stance Push Up (Wide Feet)
Muscles Worked: Chest, Triceps, Abdominals, Shoulders, Legs

How to:
1. Place one single push up bar in alignment with your right shoulder in a vertical position. Grab the one bar with your right hand and elevate your upper body in the air with your right arm fully extended up. Position your legs on the bench, spread them out wide, and stand on the balls of your feet. Place your left hand behind your back. Make sure your body is fully extended and your lower back and butt are straight at all times. This is your starting position.

2. While breathing in, engage your core, then slowly lower your body straight down until your face is about 3-4 inches off the floor. Your body should be in the decline position at this point. Pause for a second at the bottom. *Note: Because of the awkward position, maintain your balance at all times.*

3. While breathing out, slowly raise your body back up to the starting position. When set is completed, switch exercise to left arm and repeat process.

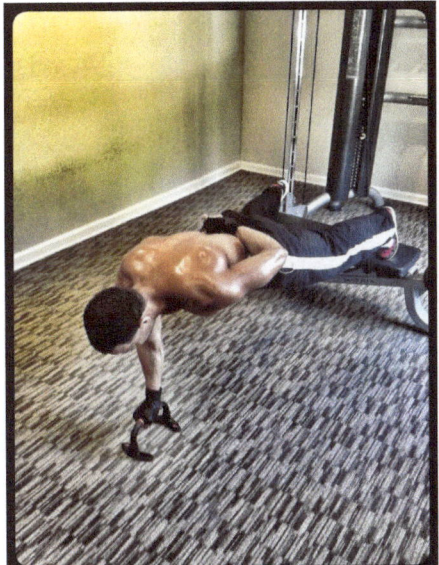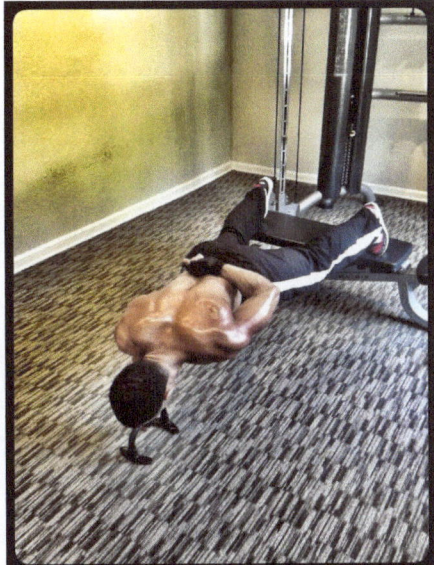

**Note: For Variations 38-40, there are 3 separate levels of advanced movements. **

Variation #38

Handstand w/ Feet On Wall Stance Push Up (Vertical)

Muscles Worked: Chest, Triceps, Abdominals, Shoulders, Legs

How to:

1. Place the push up bars in a vertical position about 12-16 inches away from the wall. Grab both bars and catapult your body up in the air in a handstand position by placing both heels of your feet up against the wall. Push your body all the way up until your arms are fully extended. Your back should be arched at this point. This is your starting position.

2. While breathing in, engage your core, then slowly lower your body straight down with the heels of your feet sliding down the wall until your head is about 1-inch off the floor. Pause for a second at the bottom. *Note: Because of the awkward position, maintain your balance at all times.*

3. While breathing out, slowly raise your body back up to the starting position.

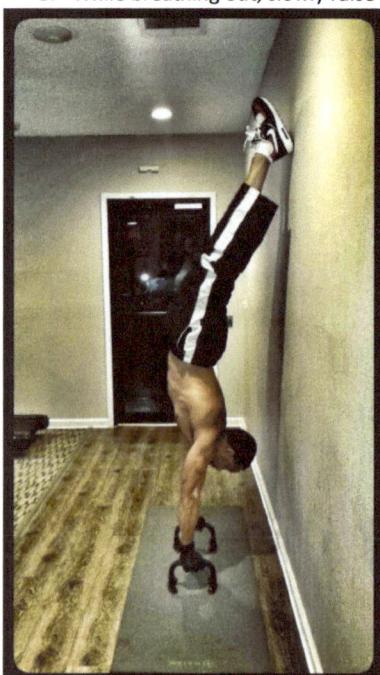 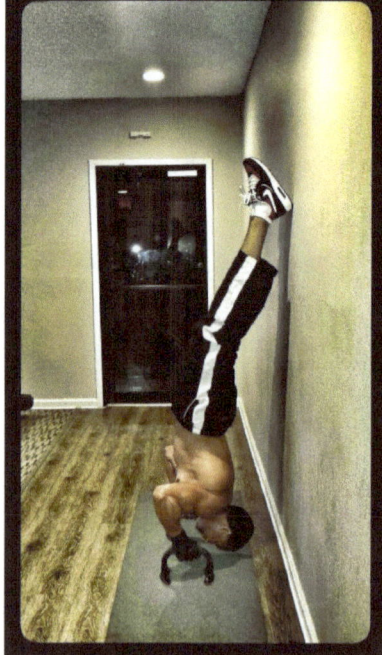

Variation #39

<u>Handstand w/ One-Foot on Wall Stance Push Up</u> (Vertical)
Muscles Worked: Chest, Triceps, Abdominals, Shoulders, Legs

How to:
1. Place the push up bars in a vertical position about 12-16 inches away from the wall. Grab both bars and catapult your body up in the air in the handstand position by placing both heels of your feet up against the wall. Push your body all the way up until your arms are fully extended. Then remove your right leg from the wall until your foot is in alignment with the push up bars. Your back should be arched at this point. This is your starting position.

2. While breathing in, engage your core, then slowly lower your body straight down with your left heel sliding down the wall and your right leg continuing to come down away from the wall until your head is about 1-inch off the floor. Pause for a second at the bottom. *Note: Because of the awkward position, maintain your balance at all times.*

3. While breathing out, slowly raise your body back up to the starting position.

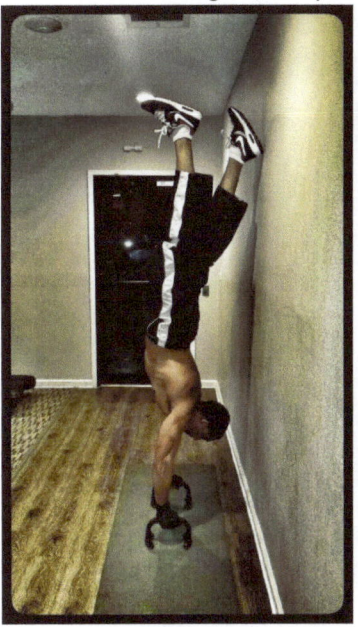 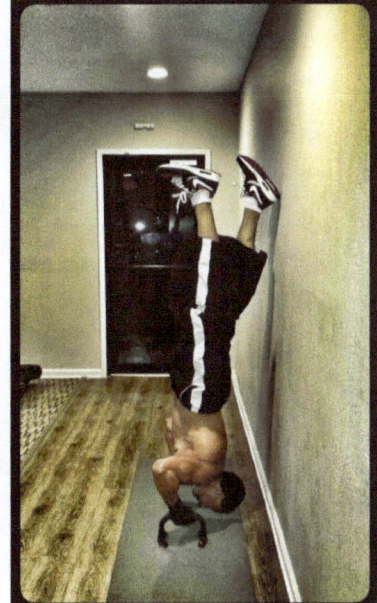

Variation #40

Handstand w/ Both Feet Off-Wall Stance Push Up (Vertical)
Muscles Worked: Chest, Triceps, Abdominals, Shoulders, Legs

How to:

1. Place the push up bars in a vertical position about 12-16 inches away from the wall. Grab both bars and catapult your body up in the air in the handstand position by placing both heels of your feet up against the wall. Push your body all the way up until your arms are fully extended. Then carefully remove both feet off the wall until your legs and feet are in alignment with the push up bars. Your back should be slightly arched with your body in a straight line at this point. This is your starting position.

2. While breathing in, engage your core, then slowly lower your body straight down in mid air until your head is about 1-inch off the floor. Pause for a second at the bottom. *Note: Because this is the most advanced movement of the 3 handstands, maintain extreme balance at all times.*

3. While breathing out, slowly raise your body back up to the starting position.

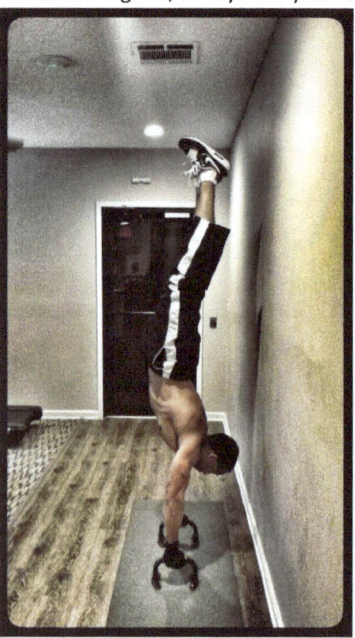 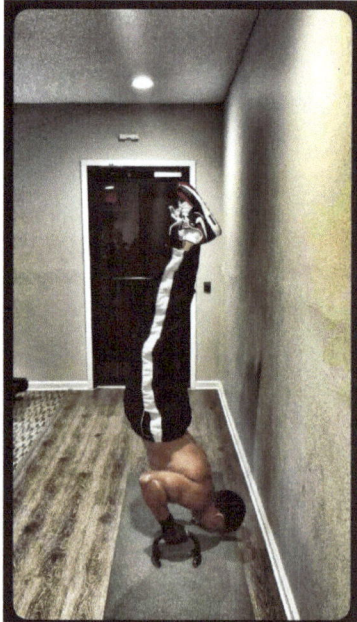

BONUS
The Push Up Bar
Ab Exercises

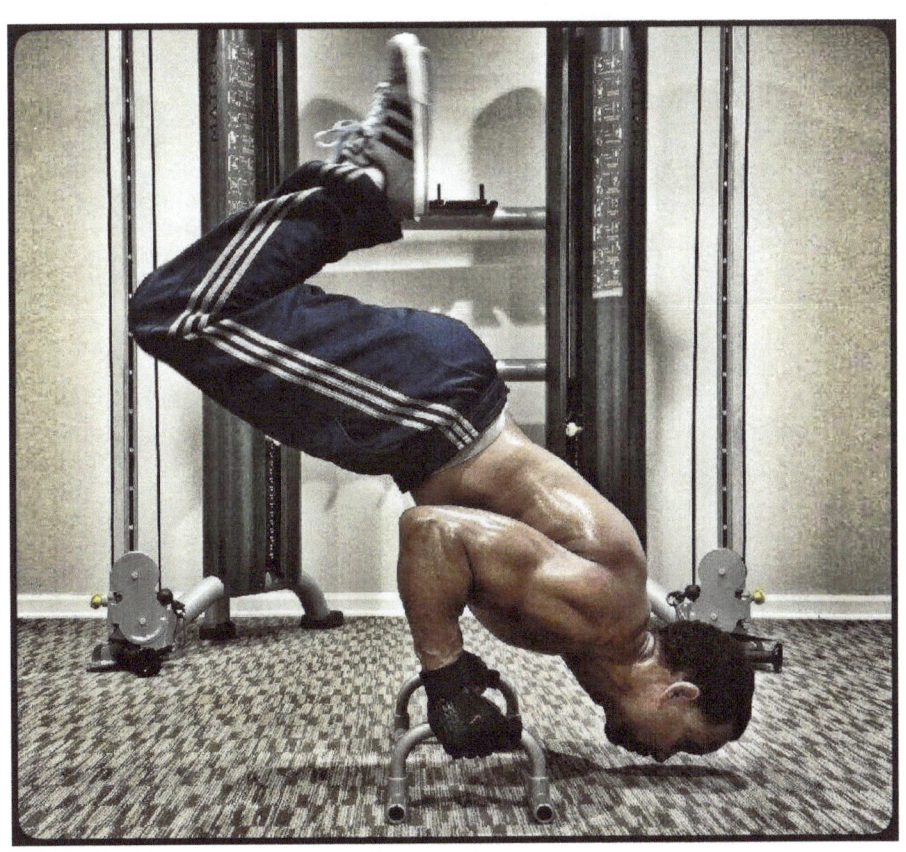

In general, when performing pushups on the push up bars correctly, you're going to feel your abs contracting like never before. Now when you isolate your core/abdominal area by performing specific ab exercises on the push up bars, your abs are going to be worked and challenged to an all new level of strength, definition, endurance, and power. As a bonus, I've also put together in this book, 12 ab exercises that you can do on the push up bars to really help maximize your core to help give your abs that sexy six-pack look. These exercises are pretty advanced; but not worry, with practice, determination, and consistency, within a few weeks, you'll be able to master these exercises with ease.

Variation #1

<u>The L-Sit Hold (Horizontal)</u>
Muscles Worked: Chest, Triceps, Abdominals, Shoulders, Legs

How to:

1. Place the push up bars about body weight apart in width in a horizontal position. Place your body in between each push up bar. Grab each bar and elevate your body in mid-air with your arms fully extended and your legs placed together fully extended out in the L-Sit position. This is your starting position.

2. While breathing in and out, engage your core, and hold the L-Sit position in mid-air for about 30-60 seconds, depending on your fitness level. (Beginners may have to hold the L-Sit position for a shorter duration.)

3. After desired time has elapsed, slowly lower your body back down.

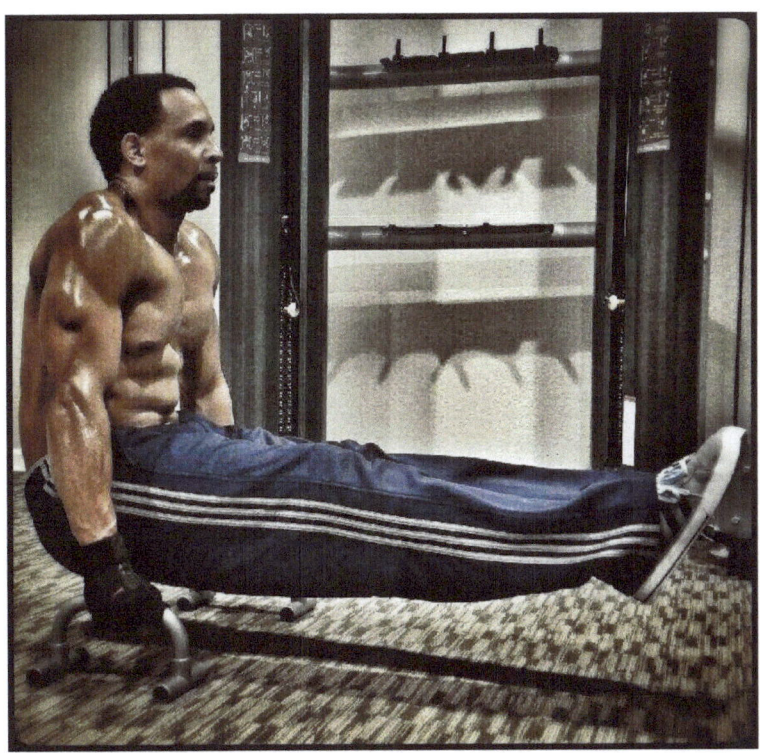

Variation #2

Tuck Leg Sit to the L-Sit (Horizontal)

Muscles Worked: Chest, Triceps, Abdominals, Shoulders, Legs

How to:

1. Place the push up bars about body weight apart in width in a horizontal position. Place your body in between each push up bar. Grab each bar and elevate your body in mid-air with your arms fully extended and your legs tucked closely together to your chest. This is your starting position.

2. While breathing in, engage your core, then fully extend your legs out and together until your body is completely in the L-Sit position. Pause for a second.

3. While breathing out, return your body slowly back to the starting position.

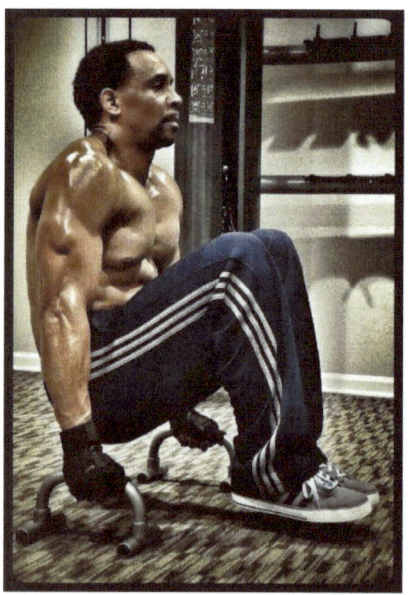
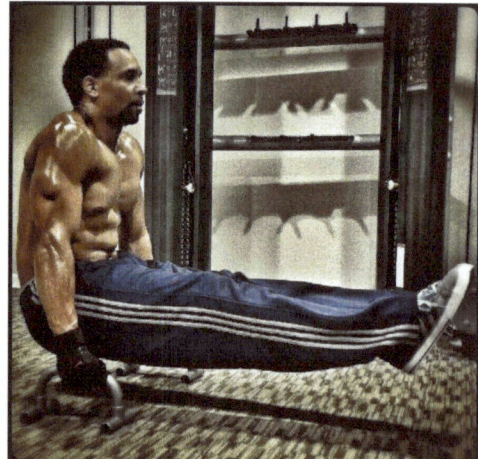

Variation #3

In and Out Leg L-Sit (Horizontal)

Muscles Worked: Chest, Triceps, Abdominals, Shoulders, Legs

How to:

1. Place the push up bars about body weight apart in width in a horizontal position. Place your body in between each push up bar. Grab each bar and elevate your body in mid-air with your arms fully extended and your legs placed together fully extended out in the L-Sit position. This is your starting position.

2. While breathing in, engage your core, then while maintaining your body in the L-Sit position, slowly open your legs as wide as you can. Hold this position for one second.

3. While breathing out, return your legs and body back to the starting position.

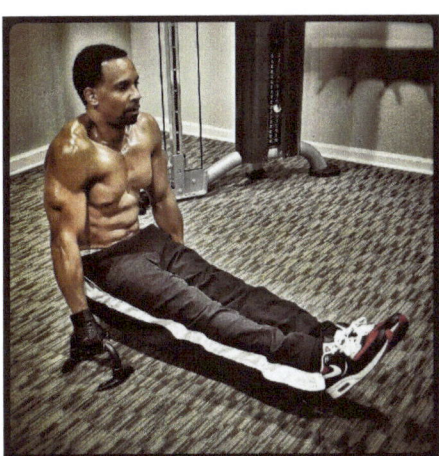 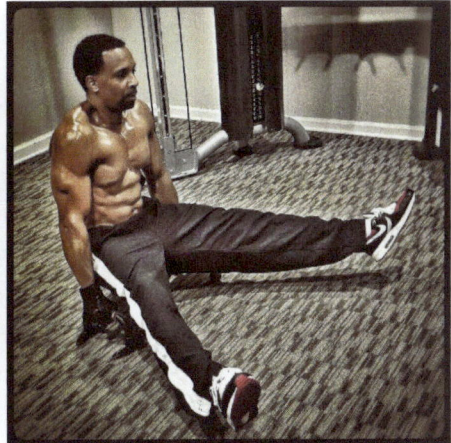

Variation #4

L-Sit Scissor Chops (Horizontal)

Muscles Worked: Chest, Triceps, Abdominals, Shoulders, Legs

How to:

1. Place the push up bars about body weight apart in width in a horizontal position. Place your body in between each push up bar. Grab each bar and elevate your body in mid-air with your arms fully extended and your legs placed together fully extended out in the L-Sit position. This is your starting position.

2. While breathing in and out, engage your core, then with a slow and controlled motion, chop your legs up and down without allowing them to come in contact with the floor.

3. When done with your desired reps, return back to the starting position.

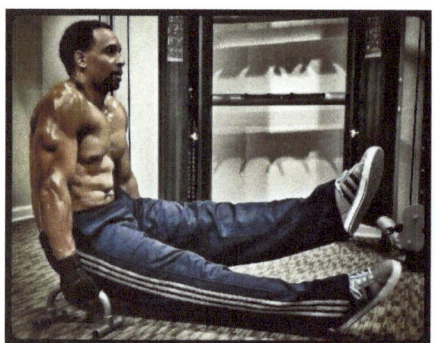 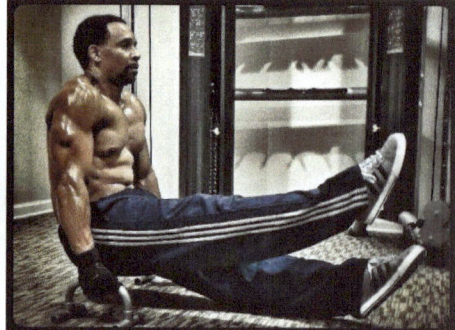

Variation #5
L-Sit Side-to-Side Swings (Horizontal)
Muscles Worked: Chest, Triceps, Abdominals, Shoulders, Legs

How to:
1. Place the push up bars about body weight apart in width in a horizontal position. Place your body in between each push up bar. Grab each bar and elevate your body in mid-air with your arms fully extended and your legs placed together fully extended out in the L-Sit position. This is your starting position.

2. While breathing in and out, engage your core, then with a slow and controlled motion, swing your legs from left to right in the L-Sit position without allowing them to come in contact with the floor.

3. When done with your desired reps, return back to the starting position.

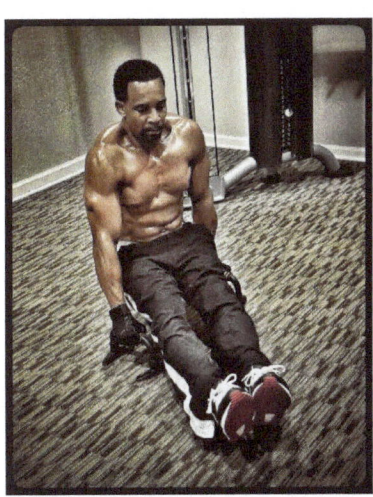
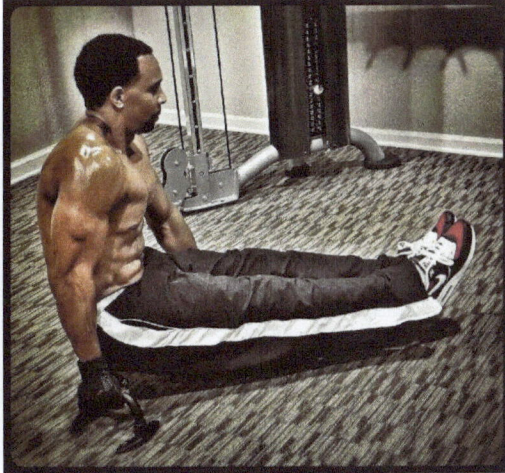

Variation #6

Tuck Alt. Leg Kick Out L-Sit (Horizontal)

Muscles Worked: Chest, Triceps, Abdominals, Shoulders, Legs

How to:

1. Place the push up bars about body weight apart in width in a horizontal position. Place your body in between each push up bar. Grab each bar and elevate your body in mid-air with your arms fully extended and your legs tucked closely together to your chest. This is your starting position.

2. While breathing in, engage your core, then slowly kick out your left leg until it is completely straight in the L-Sit position. Make sure your right leg remains bent and tucked towards your chest area. Both legs remain off the floor during the entire duration of the exercise. Pause for a second once your left leg is fully extended out.

3. While breathing out, slowly return your left leg back to the starting position. Alternate leg and repeat process.

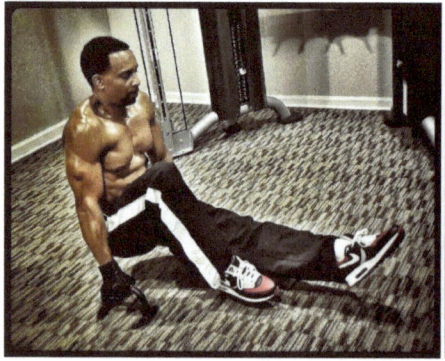 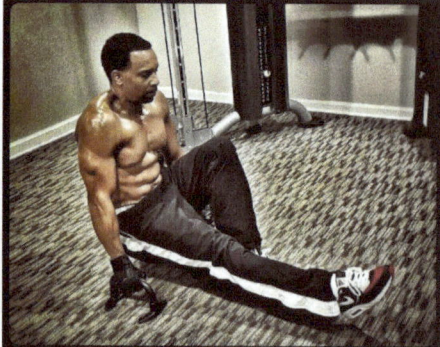

Variation #7

L-Sit to the V-Up (Horizontal)

Muscles Worked: Chest, Triceps, Abdominals, Shoulders, Legs

How to:

1. Place the push up bars about body weight apart, in width, in a horizontal position. Place your body in between each push up bar. Grab each bar and elevate your body in mid-air with your arms fully extended and your legs placed together fully extended out in the L-Sit position. This is your starting position.

2. While breathing in, engage your core, then slowly raise both legs up to the "V-Up" position. Pause for a second at the top of the movement.

3. While breathing out, slowly return your body back to the starting position.

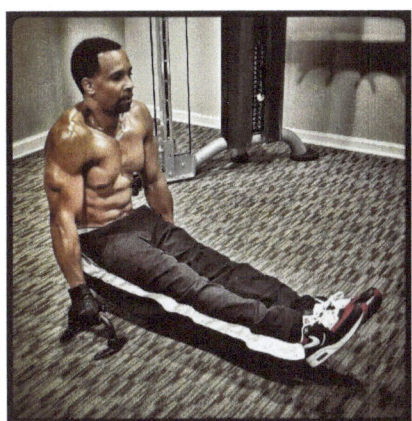 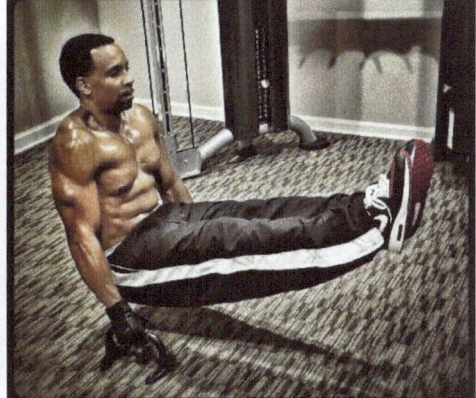

Variation #8

L-Sit Criss-Cross (Horizontal)

Muscles Worked: Chest, Triceps, Abdominals, Shoulders, Legs

How to:

1. Place the push up bars about body weight apart, in width, in a horizontal position. Place your body in between each push up bar. Grab each bar and elevate your body in mid-air with your arms fully extended and your legs placed together fully extended out in the L-Sit position. This is your starting position.

2. While breathing in and out, engage your core, then slowly start criss-crossing your legs one over top of the other while remaining in the L-Sit position. Your body remains off the floor during the entire duration of the exercise.

3. When desired reps are completed, return your body back to the starting position.

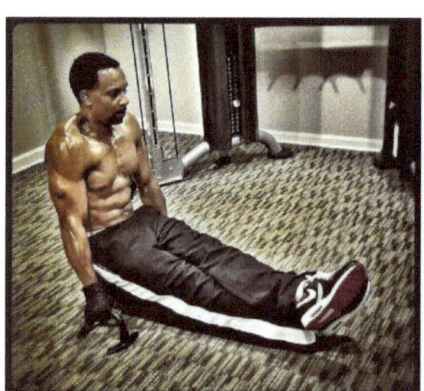 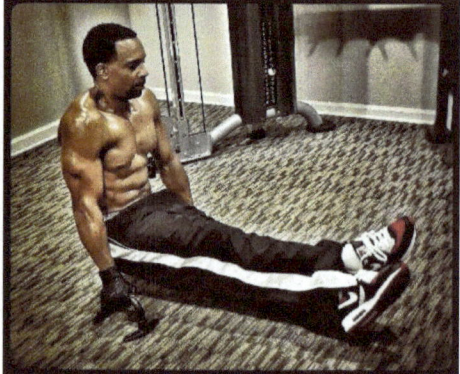

Variation #9

Tuck Planche Hold (Horizontal)

Muscles Worked: Chest, Triceps, Abdominals, Shoulders, Legs

How to:
1. Place the push up bars about body weight apart, in width, in a horizontal position. Place your body in between each push up bar. Raise your body up into the tuck planche position with your knees and legs behind you. Your body should be elevated about 2-3 inches off the floor. This is your starting position.

2. While breathing in and out, engage your core, and hold the tuck planche position for about 30 seconds to one minute, depending on your fitness level. (Beginners may have to hold the tuck planche position for a shorter duration.)

3. After desired time has elapsed, slowly lower your body back down.

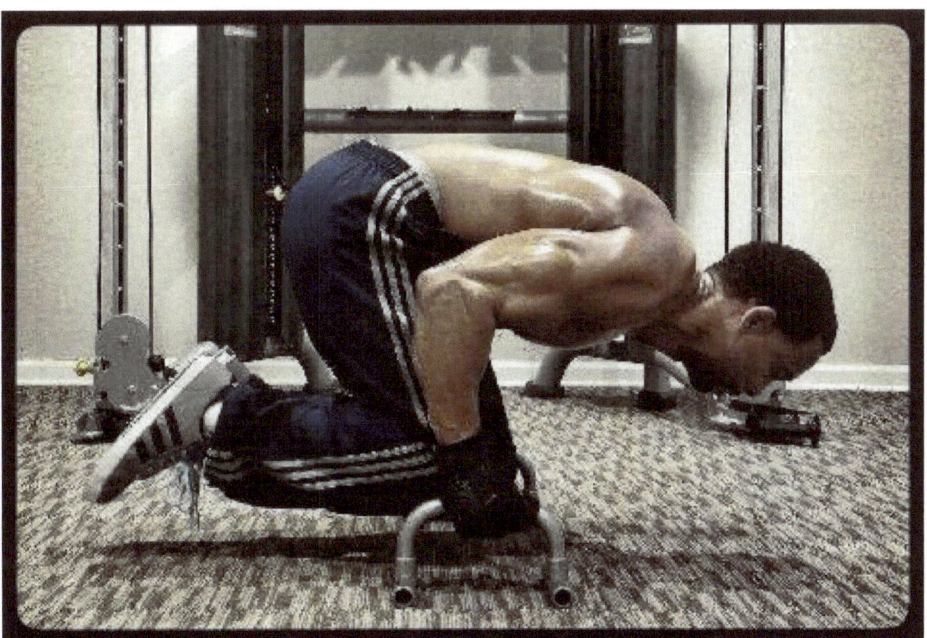

Variation #10

<u>Tuck Planche Hold to the Superman Nose Dive (Horizontal)</u>
Muscles Worked: Chest, Triceps, Abdominals, Shoulders, Legs

How to:

1. Place the push up bars about body weight apart, in width, in a horizontal position. Place your body in between each push up bar. Raise your body up into the tuck planche position with your knees and legs behind you. Your body should be elevated about 2-3 inches off the floor. This is your starting position.

2. While breathing in, engage your core, then slowly and carefully raise your legs back and up until your body is at a 45-degree angle with your nose being 1-inch off the floor. Hold this position for one second. (*Note: Maintain good balance at all times.*)

3. While breathing out, slowly and carefully bring your body back down to the starting position.

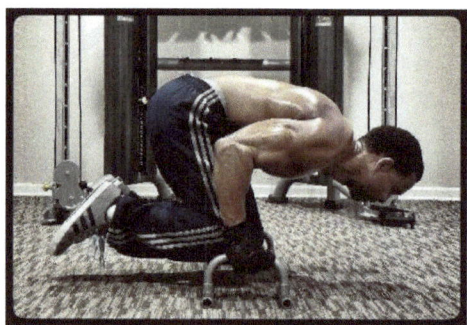

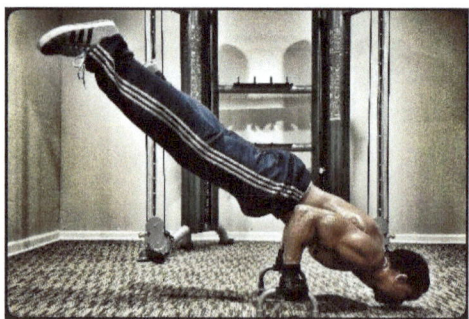

Variation #11

Scorpion Crunch (Horizontal)

Muscles Worked: Chest, Triceps, Abdominals, Shoulders, Legs

How to:

1. Place the push up bars about body weight apart, in width, in a horizontal position. Place your body in between each push up bar. Raise your body up into the tuck planche position with your knees and legs behind you. Your body should be elevated about 2-3 inches off the floor. This is your starting position.

2. While breathing in, engage your core, then slowly and carefully raise your tucked legs up and back behind you until your body forms a "scorpion tail". Hold that position for one second at the top. (*Note: Maintain good balance at all times.*)

3. While breathing out, slowly and carefully bring your body back down to the starting position.

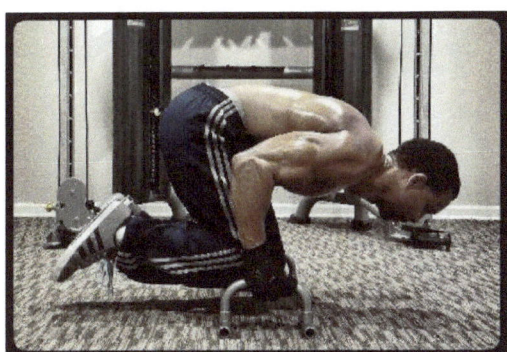 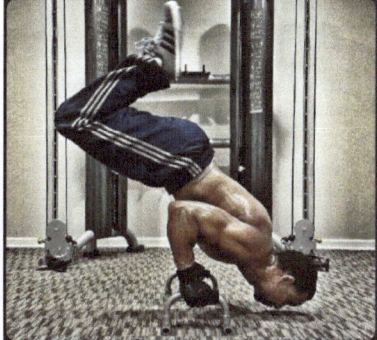

Variation #12

Scorpion to the Superman Nose Dive (Horizontal)

Muscles Worked: Chest, Triceps, Abdominals, Shoulders, Legs

How to:

1. Place the push up bars about body weight apart, in width, in a horizontal position. Place your body in between each push up bar. Elevate your body until you're in the tuck planche position, then continue to raise your body to the "scorpion" position. This is your starting position.

2. While breathing in, engage your core, then slowly and carefully from the "scorpion" position, straighten your bent legs out until they're completely straight and your body forms a 45-degree angle, with your nose being 1-inch off the floor. Hold this position for one second. (*Note: Maintain good balance at all times.*)

3. While breathing out, slowly and carefully bring your legs back to the "scorpion" position.

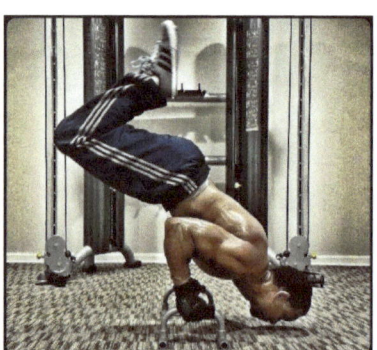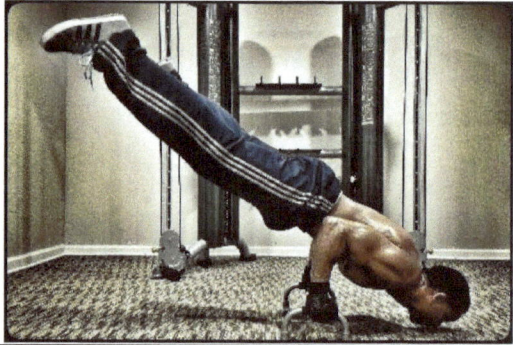

The Workouts

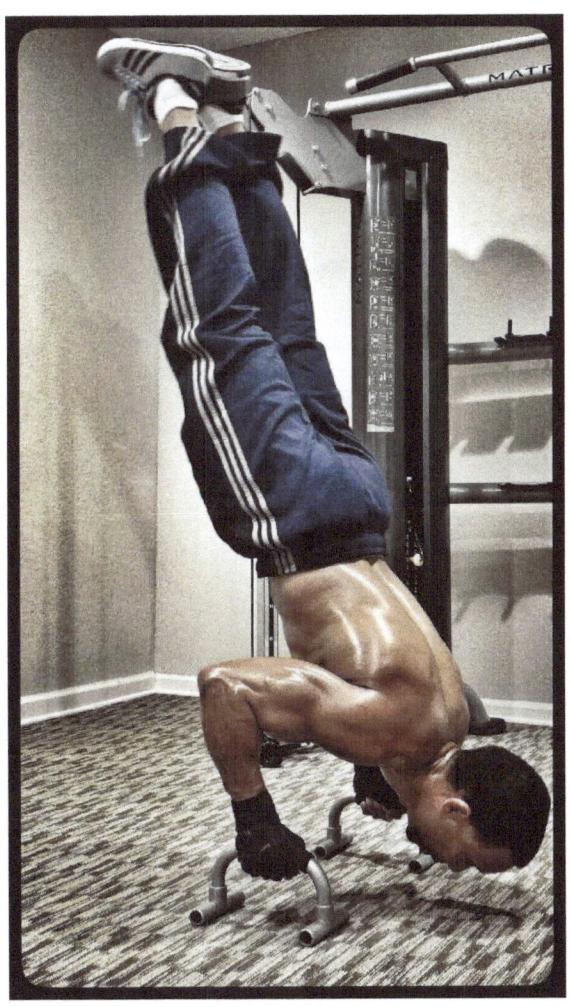

Standard Style

For Variation Numbers 1-8

Level 1	Level 2	Level 3
3-4 sets of 5-7 reps	5-7 sets of 8-10 reps	8-10 sets of 11-15 reps

Intermediate Style

For Variation Numbers 9-22

Level 1	Level 2	Level 3
5-6 sets of 6-8 reps	7-8 sets of 10-12 reps	9-10 sets of 13-15 reps

Advanced Style

For Variation Numbers 23-40

Level 1	Level 2	Level 3
7-8 sets of 8-10 reps	9-10 sets of 13-15 reps	11-15 sets of 16-20 reps

Bonus Abs

For Variation Numbers 1 & 9

Standard Level	Intermediate Level	Advanced Level
3-4 sets of 20-25 sec holds	5-7 sets of 30-40 sec holds	8-10 sets of 45-60 sec holds

For Variation Numbers 2-8, 10-12

Standard Level	Intermediate Level	Advanced Level
7-8 sets of 8-10 reps	9-10 sets of 12-15 reps	11-15 sets of 16-20 reps

Conclusion

Throughout this book, I've shared with you the effectiveness, advantages, and greatness of taking your physique to a whole new level by using the pushup bars. For more than 10 years, I've incorporated the pushup bars in my daily workout regimens. As a result, my strength, endurance, power and overall build is at an all-time high...and there's still room for growth!

As a personal trainer for more than 15 years now, I truly understand the importance of callisthenic exercises for the ultimate development of your body. Doing pushups on your hands is a great callisthenic body weight exercise in itself. However, when you add the pushup bars to the mix, your outcome will be at least five times better than before.

Once again, I hope and pray that this workout book has been a blessing to you and your future workout goals. May God bless you in your quest of being the best you can be.

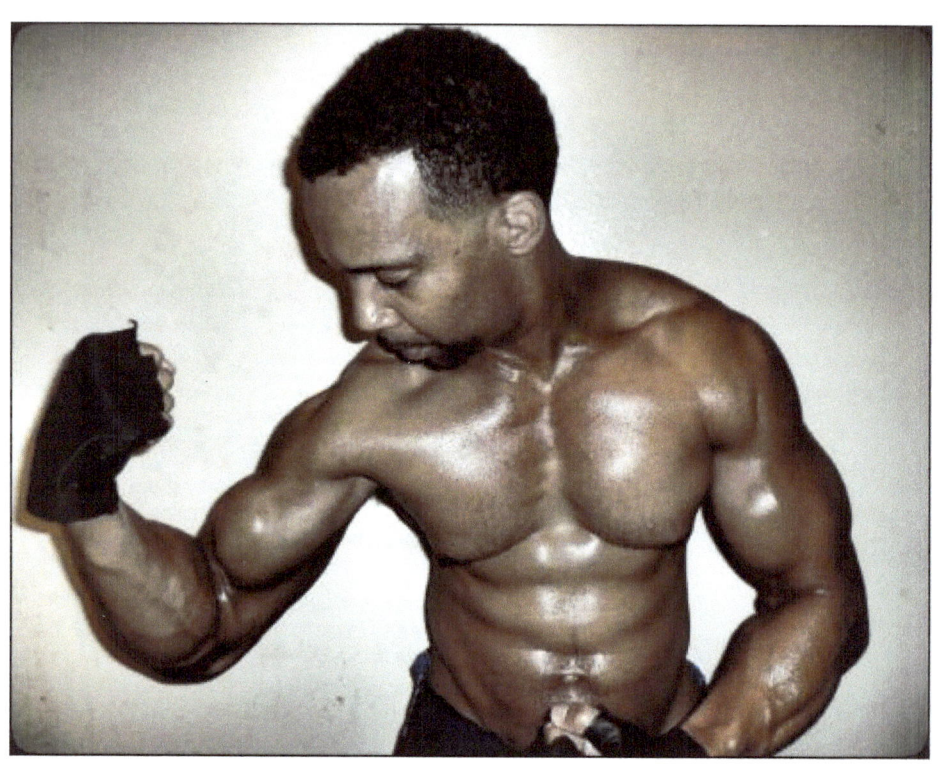

www.ingramcontent.com/pod-product-compliance
Lightning Source LLC
Chambersburg PA
CBHW050812290526
45792CB00001B/86